Extraordinary Healers

CURE Readers Honor Oncology Nurses

Volume 4

Extraordinary Healers

CURE Readers Honor Oncology Nurses

Volume 4

curemedia**group**

Dallas, Texas

Made possible with financial support from Amgen, Inc.

Published by
CURE Media Group
3102 Oak Lawn, Suite 610
Dallas, Texas 75219
www.curetoday.com

Information presented is not intended as a substitute for the personalized professional advice given by your health care provider. This publication was produced by CURE Media Group. The views expressed in this publication are not necessarily those of the publisher. Although great care has been taken to ensure accuracy, CURE Media Group and its servants or agents shall not be responsible or in any way liable for the continued currency of the information or for any errors, omissions, or inaccuracies in this book, whether arising from negligence or otherwise or for any consequences arising there from. The intention of this book is not to provide specific medical advice; therefore, all references to specific commercial products have been removed. Essays have also been edited for grammar, style, length, and clarity. Review and creation of content is solely the responsibility of CURE Media Group.

Any mention of retail products does not constitute an endorsement by the authors or the publisher.

Library of Congress Control Number: 2010940527

ISBN 978-0-980130850

Edited by Lena Huang
Designed by Susan Douglass
Layout/Photo Coordination by Glenn Zamora
Event Coordination by Alexandra Hurd

Printed in the United States of America

This book is dedicated to all oncology nurses who bring hope and healing to cancer patients and their loved ones.

If you would like to give this book as a gift to your Extraordinary Healer, we've provided this page for your message.

This book honors:

_____

_____

_____

_____

_____

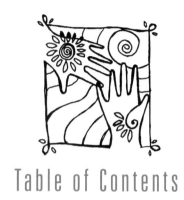

Table of Contents

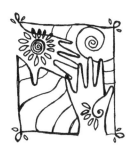

The Evolution of Oncology Nurses

BEFORE THERE WERE ONCOLOGY NURSES, there were nurses drawn to care for cancer patients. They faced barriers, such as the commonly held belief that cancer was a terminal disease, and thus patients should not be told they have the disease. And they were on the forefront of radium therapy, which had many nurses handling the toxic substances without knowing the dangers.

Nursing texts early in the 20th century advised those caring for cancer patients to "be a source of strength and security for the patient."

It wasn't until 1947 that the first university course on cancer nursing was organized to respond to, as *The New York Times* story said, "The increasing national demand for nurses specializing in cancer treatment and prevention." The course was funded by a grant from the American Cancer Society New York Division.

One nurse, Virginia Barckley, who was an advocate for specializing cancer nursing, came back at critics of the profession with: "When revulsion is replaced by compassion, when we think, 'what can I do to help?' instead of 'Poor me!' we are functioning on a high level."

THE PROFESSIONAL ONCOLOGY NURSE

P.J. Haylock, PhD, RN, a cancer care consultant who has written on the evolution of oncology nursing, says the Nurse Training Act of 1964, a component of Lyndon Johnson's Great Society, was a catalyst for the move toward the founding of many specialty nursing organizations in the 1970s.

As clinical trials for new drugs began to increase in the 1960s, so did the need for nurses trained as data

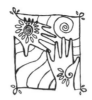

collectors for the physicians, a role that, according to Haylock, eventually expanded to serving as the liaison between clinical investigators and other disciplines in cancer care. This "team" approach began to take hold as a best practice, and nurses in cancer began further specializing in areas such as radiation, detection, patient education, nursing education, and research.

In 1975, 226 charter members formed the Oncology Nursing Society (ONS), a number that has grown to more than 37,000 today. During the past 35 years, ONS has been instrumental in the professional growth of oncology nursing, drafting standards of care and in 1979, publishing *Outcome Standards for Cancer Nursing Practice* with the American Nurses Association. Through the years, ONS has published other documents representing consensus of desired outcomes with regard to physical, psychosocial, and spiritual aspects of cancer care as ONS has become the standard bearer for the oncology nursing profession.

Today's oncology nurses work with a great deal of autonomy in a wide variety of roles and settings inside and outside of hospitals where they work "with" instead of "for" physicians.

Haylock says that just as survivors are counseled to find the "new normal" in their lives after cancer, so too are oncology nurses learning these new realities to integrate into the delivery of cancer care.

"Cancer nurses have come such a long way, and are still finding their way in the new normal of their professional duties," Haylock says. "Today's oncology nurses work with a great deal of autonomy in a wide variety of roles and settings inside and outside of hospitals where they work 'with' instead of 'for' physicians."

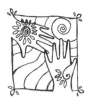

The role of the oncology nurse researchers, Haylock says, has been to explore interventions relating to all aspects of physical and emotional coping.

"Most notably," Haylock says, "oncology nursing as a discipline is searching for ways to accommodate the evolving cancer survivor populations, to include knowing about and planning for late and long-term effects of cancer and cancer treatment, and the needs of people who live with treatable-but-not-curable cancers."

THE FUTURE ONCOLOGY NURSE

The evolution of the oncology nurse can be seen in the expanded roles and responsibilities nurses assume today. Oncology nurse managers search for cost-effective means to meet the needs of patients in a particular setting, including staff numbers and legal scope of practice. Oncology nurse navigators guide patients through every aspect of diagnosis, treatment, and survivorship while others have attained new levels of education that elevate their roles and responsibilities into areas of the clinical nurse specialist and the nurse practitioner. These advanced practice nurses work alongside physicians and other members of the health care team to provide a multidisciplinary approach to health and well-being for cancer patients and cancer survivors.

The new goals for attainable health care hold promise for even greater professionalism as oncology nurses have moved into national decision-making and policy roles.

In October 2010, the Institute of Medicine released *The Future of Nursing: Leading Change, Advancing Health.* This report, funded by the Robert Wood Johnson Foundation and the Institute of Medicine, is the result of a two-year initiative to assess and transform the nursing profession. It identifies four key messages for the future of nursing and its more than three million members, the largest segment of the nation's health care workforce.

First, it calls for nurses to practice to the full extent of their education and training and points specifically

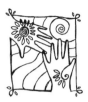

at advanced practice registered nurses who, depending on state nurse practice acts, may or may not be able to perform at the level their education offers.

Second, nurses should obtain higher levels of education and training through an improved teaching system. This speaks to the expanding roles of nurses to master technological tools and information management systems while collaborating and coordinating care across teams of health professionals. "Nurses also should be educated with physicians and other health professionals both as students and throughout their careers in lifelong learning opportunities," the report explains.

Third, nurses must be included, along with other health care professionals, in "any redesign efforts" of health care in the United States. This requires that nurses not only participate in but lead decision-making efforts for change at every level.

Fourth, additional research and information is needed to improve the infrastructure needed to support the changing role of the oncology nurse. The report states, "Once an improved infrastructure for collecting and analyzing workforce data is in place, systematic assessment and projection of workforce requirements by role, skill mix, region, and demographics will be needed to inform changes in nursing practice and education."

For oncology nursing this means an ever greater impact on those on the cancer journey.

—Kathy LaTour, *CURE*'s editor-at-large

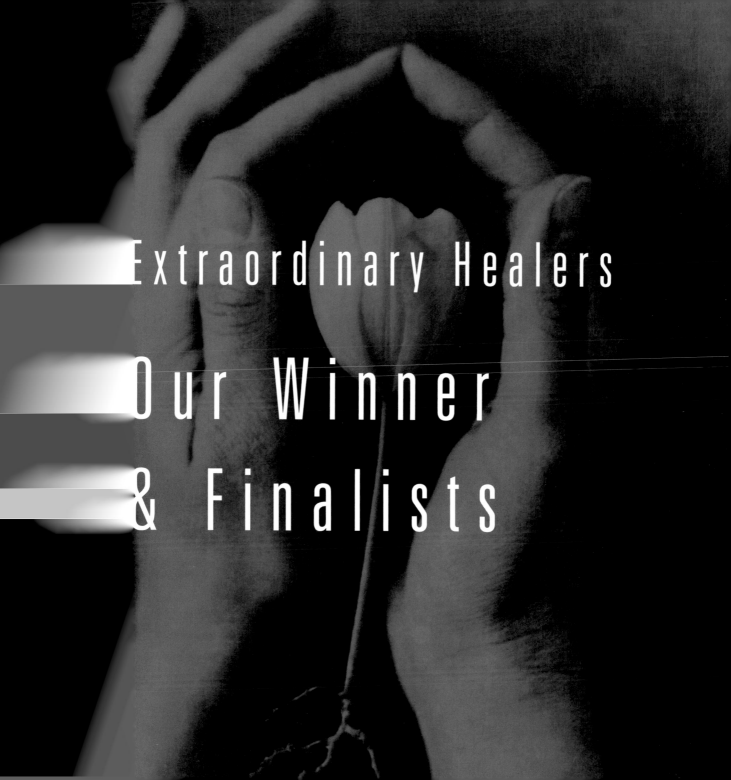

Extraordinary Healers

Our Winner
& Finalists

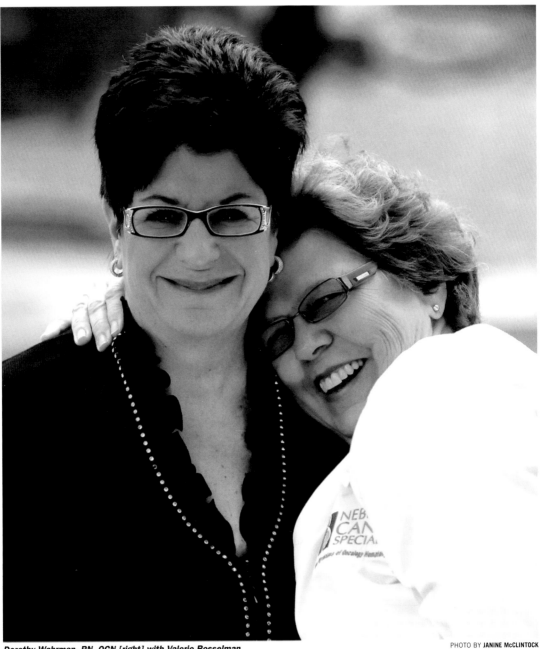

Dorothy Wahrman, RN, OCN [right] with Valerie Bosselman

PHOTO BY JANINE McCLINTOCK

Beginning to End

WINNER OF THE 2010 EXTRAORDINARY HEALER AWARD FOR ONCOLOGY NURSING

DOROTHY WAHRMAN, RN, OCN [NEBRASKA CANCER SPECIALISTS IN OMAHA, NEBRASKA]

WRITTEN BY VALERIE BOSSELMAN

SHE WAS THERE in the beginning.

THE FIRST DAY of chemo. While my daughter and I were veterans of the Methodist Estabrook Cancer Center, December 27, 2006, marked the start of full-scale chemo and radiation. My beautiful girl was no longer in remission from adrenal cortical carcinoma but was in the fight for her life. ACC is rare, aggressive, and often fatal within five years.

We remembered the bewildered feeling in 2004, right after Megan's college graduation, when we learned she had cancer. However, 18 months of glorious remission and Megan's youthful optimism had lulled us into a state that no longer imagined the worst. Regretfully, our 2006 fall lineup included adrenal cancer that had metastasized in three abdominal locations, the removal of her left kidney, and a laminectomy to remove a paralyzing spinal tumor. The news that cancer had advanced on Megan's lungs came just in time for Christmas. The worst was upon us.

I was always resolute in knowing Megan was receiving the best medical care imaginable. After all, Dr. Robert Langdon was not only her oncologist but also our next-door neighbor and the father of six girls. He loved my girl like his own. I never doubted that every decision—including his selection of Dorothy Wahrman as Megan's chemo nurse—would be the best.

My intuition did not disappoint. In our first meeting with Dorothy, Megan sat in what would become her all-too-familiar leather recliner; I sat as close as possible to her. We were so afraid. Dorothy pulled up a rolling stool and took us from fear to familiar—from feeling forgotten by God to a new family of health care professionals. She wheeled right into our hearts, and the stack of printed material she presented seemed unimportant. I knew she would be a guide and translator for the uncertain days ahead.

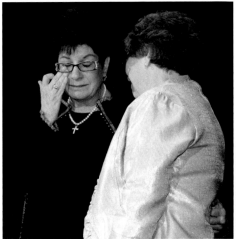

Dorothy Wahrman, RN, OCN [right] with Valerie Bosselman at the 2010 Extraordinary Healer Award ceremony.

She was there in the middle.

Chemo became routine, and we found a new normal. Our daily visit to the cancer center included a bag loaded with one of her "woobies" (code for a favorite blanket) and a laptop for web surfing to keep Megan up to date on the latest fashions. Dorothy oversaw the complicated chemo protocol—a $10,000-a-month clinical trial—while chatting with my girl about the latest star gossip and delivering snacks prepared for Megan the night before. She would polish off moments by pulling the woobie up over Megan's shoulders, making sure she wasn't cold. Dorothy would ask Megan, "Do I cut my hair short or not?" and my hairless girl would tell Dorothy how fabulous a new "do" would be in her convertible with the top down and a breeze blowing through her hair. Oh, how Megan wanted hair. And, oh, how she loved Dorothy.

Dorothy was also part of the magnificent team that orchestrated Megan's dream night with Justin Timberlake. Megan's oncology team became her personal Make a Wish Foundation and gave her the night of her life. Megan said, "I'd rather have 30 minutes of wonderful than a lifetime of nothing special." The team delivered not only the superstar, but also his personal trainer, Jason, who escorted Megan for the evening.

It was a once-upon-a-time evening, but since life is not always storybook, Dorothy was also there when Megan's white blood counts were at deadly levels. She was there before hospice, when the pain was so severe we would be at the cancer center door when they opened for the next blast of morphine. She was there when the trial study succeeded, there when it failed, and there when the sun was shining. She was also there for a sobbing mom waiting for valet parking in the rain without an umbrella because the parking garage was under construction.

She was there in the end.

On March 17, 2008, Megan was moved from home to Josie Harper Hospice House. On March 21, Good Friday, the hospice team scrambled for solutions to manage Megan's excruciating pain. Cancer seized my daughter's body; the spinal tumors left her in agony. Even with staggering levels of narcotics, pain management was nearly impossible. God have mercy.

Mid-morning on Good Friday, Dorothy left her oncology station to drive to Hospice House to see Megan for the last time. She just knew to come. Dorothy later wrote me in an e-mail:

> *I truly cannot say why I chose to go see Megan on Good Friday. Something inside me drew me there that day. I guess I knew that things were bad, and Megan's time on earth was short … When I arrived I saw and felt the suffering of Megan and her family and wished there was something more I could do for all of them. I could only pray that God would give them all the strength that they would need.*

What Dorothy didn't know was that paperwork was in motion to place Megan into a drug-induced sleep to manage her erratic pain. We were just hours away from our last words with my girl. How did Dorothy know right when to come? I must say that, in all my months with this most remarkable woman, her ability to sense the every need of patient and family was the most beautiful and natural part of her character. I can still see Dorothy, sitting on the edge of Megan's bed, boldly swooping my beautiful girl into her arms and tenderly cradling her frail frame. So motherly in her stature, it appeared she was pressing Megan tightly into her bosom, but in reality she was pressing my girl into her heart for the last time.

Dorothy silently held Megan's hand and then told her goodbye. My daughter was not healed in any physical way. But Dorothy Wahrman gave us peace by holding our hand from beginning to end. That's what makes her an extraordinary healer. ❧

Defining Moment in Nursing: A Calling

BY DOROTHY WAHRMAN, RN, OCN

I BEGAN MY career in the mid-1970s when oncology nursing was just beginning to be recognized as a specialty.

I WAS ON the medical/surgical floor at the hospital when the hospital decided to add an outpatient oncology unit and one of the doctors asked me to work for him. It was a "chance" that I ended up in the field I love, where I know I can make a difference in the lives of patients.

Over the years, I came to understand that my career was a calling, not a job—a point that has been driven home many times. But one family stands out in my mind.

I had stopped in to check on a woman and her husband who were new to cancer. She had been diagnosed with breast cancer, and when I met her and her husband, I could see the fear in both their eyes. I was chatting with the wife, making a connection, and noticed she shared an unusual last name with a man I had treated years before at another institution.

I asked if she knew the man, only to find out that it was her father-in-law—her husband's father. I told them how I remember seeing him at Christmas after his treatment had ended. He showed up with a poinsettia that was as big as he was. It was an annual event for him until his death.

The couple couldn't believe I remembered him when it had been more than 10 years since his death. Later, the woman's husband told me that knowing I had cared for his father had made such a difference. He said I was the sign that he was there for them, and his wife would be fine. It was a powerful affirmation.

To this day, I still get a poinsettia every Christmas, but it never says who it's from.

It's events like this when a patient comes back to look me up when treatment has ended that reminds me that I made a difference in people's lives—and that is why what I do is more than a job. It's a calling. ❧

My Partner in Recovery

FINALIST FOR THE 2010 EXTRAORDINARY HEALER AWARD FOR ONCOLOGY NURSING

JACKIE BROADWAY-DUREN, MSN, FNP-BC [M.D. ANDERSON CANCER CENTER IN HOUSTON, TEXAS]

WRITTEN BY CATHERINE GILMORE

IT IS HARD to know where to begin in describing Jackie. I will start by saying that five years ago when I was first diagnosed with leukemia, I chose M.D. Anderson for my care because of its reputation. I expected to get excellent treatment, and I have not been disappointed.

HAVING SAID that, Jackie exceeded even my very high expectations. She is enormously competent and talented. In the complicated business of being a cancer patient, often you don't know what you don't know. Jackie anticipates that very situation and volunteers information in a comprehensive and understandable context. Her exceptional knowledge enables her to not only respond just to the question asked, but she goes further to help the patient fully understand implications and options. She has the ability to deliver difficult information in a way that is honest and clear but compassionate. She is always sure to balance the challenges ahead with a quiet, positive view that lays out solutions and a plan. It is always clear that we are in this fight together and everything possible will be done to win.

I am old enough and have had enough health challenges to be a very experienced health care consumer. I know good care from poor, and Jackie is in a category of her own. She is incredibly responsive and nothing is ever too much trouble. No call or e-mail is undeserving of immediate action. She forms a personal bond with patients and always seems to understand the issues that make them unique. She is the very definition of patient advocate.

My best interests are always her first priority. Although there are many examples, the first came while I was at M.D. Anderson for a checkup and needed treatment. Jackie asked me when I wanted to start. I said I

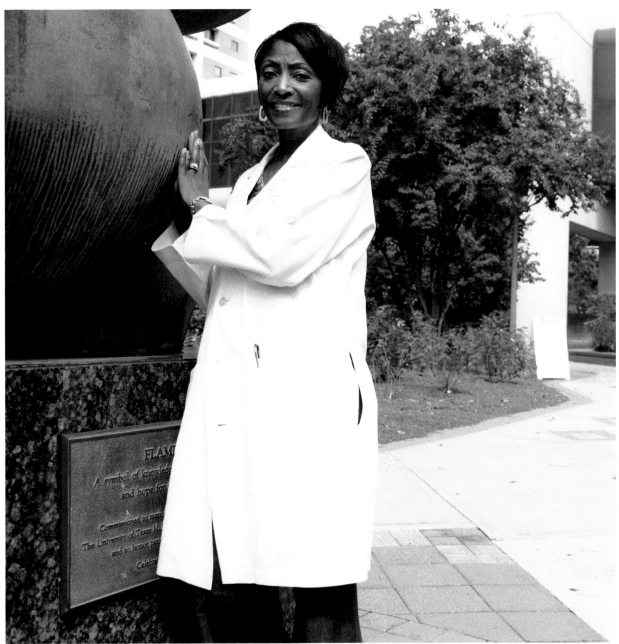

Jackie Broadway-Duren, MSN, FNP-BC

wish I could start today but whenever they could schedule me was fine. She immediately picked up the phone and was able to arrange an infusion appointment three hours later. She knows I live in Arizona and have to travel to Houston for my appointments. As always, my preferences and convenience were her top priority. This doesn't happen by magic. It takes commitment, significant effort, and a strong relationship with other organizations to make this work. I am quite amazed at Jackie's ability to engage colleagues beyond Dr. Keating's staff to augment the "team," and I know it is due to their respect and genuine admiration for her talent.

One of the most important aspects of being a patient is confidence that the entire care team is working together. Jackie and Dr. Keating clearly are a team. Being a real team—not just people who work together—is not something you see every day. The relationship she has with her colleagues is remarkable.

One of the most extraordinary examples is one I truly didn't appreciate at the time. I had chosen not to tell my mother and young nephews I had leukemia and needed treatment. My father had died of cancer, and it was a long, difficult death.

Many people have an opinion on my choice. Not only did Jackie respect and never judge in any way that decision, she focused every effort on making what I now know was an unreasonable request work—against all odds.

TEACHING MOMENT:

I am quite amazed at Jackie's ability to engage colleagues beyond Dr. Keating's staff to augment the "team," and I know it is due to their respect and genuine admiration for her talent.

13

As part of a clinical trial, I needed an infusion during the Thanksgiving holiday. I was in Boston celebrating the holiday with my family and would have had to fly to Houston or Arizona on Thanksgiving to receive treatment on Friday. It would have been impossible to explain my absence. I asked Jackie if I could get the treatment in Boston. Through her extraordinary efforts, I was treated at Dana-Farber that Friday while everyone thought I was shopping with my sister for the day. I look back on that time now and realize how much work this request took. There was only one authorized location for the clinical trial in Boston. I had no doctor in Boston and would only be a patient for one day. In spite of this, Jackie found a doctor—and not just any doctor but a specialist in leukemia—to take me as a patient, examine and clear me for treatment, and then arrange treatment all on the Friday after Thanksgiving—all without ever indicating just how hard this was to accomplish. Never once did she reveal just how impossible a request this was. I came to realize this when the infusion staff at Dana-Farber all knew I was the "special" patient. I look back and realize it would have been easier to ask her to make the sun rise in the west and set in the east.

In a world of political correctness, she and Dr. Keating start and end every appointment by hugging the patient and anyone else who is in the room. I have often joked with friends and family that, if all the chemo and treatments don't work, I believe they will hug me well. On her voicemail she ends with, "Have a blessed day." She actually means it. She never discusses her religious beliefs, rather she treats every person with respect, genuine concern, and as if they are the most important part of her day—all while making it look easy.

As I read over this nomination, I fear my attempt to describe how truly extraordinary she is falls far short of reality. I realize that, in part, it is my own limitation as a writer, but it is also her modest, inspirational, and very effective way of making everything work without ever pointing out just how remarkable a job she is doing. When people ask me why I don't worry or obsess about having leukemia, I tell them I have the best team on earth worrying for me and working every day to make sure I not only survive but thrive. Jackie is very much the face of this effort and my partner in recovery. ❧

Defining Moment in Nursing: Changing the Journey

BY JACKIE BROADWAY-DUREN, MSN, FNP-BC

IT'S KNOWING that I can do something to make a difference in the cancer journey that reminds me why I am an oncology nurse.

I KNOW oncology nursing is about medical care, but sometimes it's more about emotional support. As a nurse practitioner in the outpatient leukemia clinic at M.D. Anderson Cancer Center in Houston, I recall moments when I could bring joy or peace to a patient as the ones that have stayed with me.

They are moments like the one when 14-year-old Heather, who was dying of leukemia, told me that her biggest wish was to meet country singer Garth Brooks. I worked with the Make a Wish Foundation and was actually standing in Heather's room one morning when I heard a commotion in the hall. I went out and saw it was Brooks. We never told her he was coming. I went back in the room and said, "Heather I know you aren't having a great day, but I think I have something that will make you feel better."

She totally forgot she was sick. She leaped out of bed, and he came and sat down next to her, and it was such a joyous moment. I'll never forget the look on her face.

But, it isn't always the joyous times I recall. I had another young patient who was only 28 and had stage 4 breast cancer. It was the end of my shift one night, and I was so looking forward to going home when one of her family members came to get me.

The young woman asked her family to leave, saying it was me she needed to talk to just then.

She told me she was going to die, and she was scared. We had talked about our faith before, and I told her not to be afraid, I would stay with her.

I sat in the recliner next to the bed until the young woman slipped into a coma. I remember she had a smile on her face, so I knew she was at peace. ❧

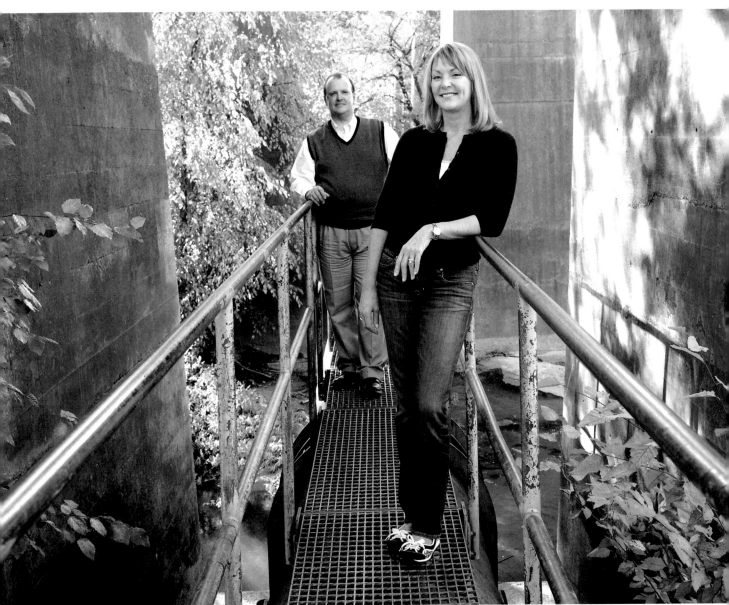

Annette Graham, ANP, AOCNP [front] with Greg Frazee

One of Cancer's Special Gifts

FINALIST FOR THE 2010 EXTRAORDINARY HEALER AWARD FOR ONCOLOGY NURSING

ANNETTE GRAHAM, ANP, AOCNP [VIRGINIA CANCER INSTITUTE IN RICHMOND, VIRGINIA]

WRITTEN BY GREG FRAZEE

AFTER FOUR DAYS of hospitalization, a needle aspiration biopsy of the newly diagnosed non-Hodgkin lymphoma tumor located in my abdomen, a PET scan, a MUGA scan, discussions about my chemotherapy treatment and the effects it would have on me, and an insertion of a power port, I was facing my final and most intimidating test. I was about to be introduced to Annette Graham. She would be administering my bone marrow biopsy.

AS I PROGRESSED through the days after my diagnosis, anxiety would overwhelm me, mostly as a result of my lack of knowledge about the procedures and processes I would be facing. Some of the tests were difficult, and in my mind, I knew they were not as difficult as the looming bone marrow biopsy.

An initial question I began asking all of the caregivers I encountered in the beginning was, "Why did you choose such a difficult profession?" I asked the question out of curiosity, and I asked it to assure myself that the person with whom I was about to interact was indeed compassionate and would understand my situation.

Annette's reply was, "I've known too many people and have been personally affected by the impact of cancer on others. I want to make their lives better."

With apologies to Dr. Seuss, the following is a recap of my first meeting with Annette Graham:

"The first time we met, I remember distinctly.

She spoke words assuring, she delivered them succinctly.

'You may feel some pain, you may feel a pinch.'

My first bone marrow biopsy, with Annette, was a cinch!"

Due to my anxiety about my first bone marrow biopsy, I did not immediately absorb the compassion and kindness contained in the person of Annette. Soon after that, I did. At our second meeting, when we started discussing the emotional impact of my recent diagnosis, I began to experience her entire skill set.

During that meeting, she asked, "Have you cried yet?" The question took me a bit by surprise. *How did she know that I wanted to?* I replied, "You know, Annette, I haven't had a good cry since I was a kid. I recognize the therapeutic relief that a good cry would provide; however, I'm a middle-aged guy. I don't do those things." She replied, "Maybe you should work on that. It would be good for you."

I knew at that very moment, we were in this as a team.

In subsequent meetings, I expressed to her that I thought some individuals, in my group of family and friends surrounding me with care and concern, were misinformed about how to talk to me and go through this process with me. She explained that none of us had done this before, and as I would need to rely on the kindness of others to support me, I needed to extend grace to them in order to help them when they stumbled through the process.

As my treatment progressed, it became apparent that I would require stem cell transplantation therapy. My chemotherapy treatments would require overnight stays in the hospital for the pre-transplantation treatments and then a three-week stay in the hospital for the stem cell treatment.

In a meeting when we discussed what was ahead of me, Annette informed me that, when any of her patients are admitted to the hospital, she gives them a "comfort gift" to take with them. The gift would be in the form of a stuffed teddy bear. I advised her that I politely disagreed with the need for me to have a "comfort gift."

"Maybe you don't," she replied, "but I feel the need to bust your chops a little bit." What could I say? I humbly accepted the gift and took it to the hospital each time I was admitted for treatment. I found myself proudly telling the story behind the gift and telling the story of the goodness of the person who gave it to me.

As I recalled the conversation in my mind, I acknowledged that Annette had indeed given me a compliment, but even more important, she had given me a challenge that I needed.

Finally, as the calendar date of my admission to the hospital for the stem cell transplantation portion of my treatment approached, my anxiety heightened. I was concerned about being treated at a large research hospital versus being accustomed to treatment in the comfortable confines of a clinic.

As I expressed my concern to Annette, she replied, "It's intimidating, I know. However, it is the best treatment for you. Furthermore, there is no doubt in my mind that you will go there and make the experience a special one for yourself and those you meet as you have done here in the clinic." I mumbled a "thank you" for her compliment. A day later, as I recalled the conversation in my mind, I acknowledged that Annette had indeed given me a compliment, but even more important, she had given me a challenge that I needed.

There are countless other anecdotes to share. When I recall them, I see Annette looking at me with compassion, understanding, challenges, camaraderie, and overwhelming kindness. I treasure the gift of her person.

"For other patients with challenges, I hope they have met,

A person of quality like my nurse, Annette." ❧

Defining Moment in Nursing: The Power of Transformation

BY ANNETTE GRAHAM, ANP, AOCNP

THE STRENGTH AND COURAGE of my patients is an inspiration to me. Soon after beginning oncology nursing, I discovered that a cancer diagnosis can also be a transforming and empowering experience.

THERE WASN'T an epiphany, per se, but one patient stands out. She was newly diagnosed with breast cancer, and I could see that she was timid and lacked self confidence. Her husband was aloof, and it was soon clear that he was not very supportive. She was so afraid. She needed extra attention, and I made sure she got it. She finished treatment and had a good prognosis.

A year later she returned for a routine follow-up. I saw her sitting in the waiting room with sunlight shining on her. She didn't look like the same woman; she was a proud lioness. In the exam room we began to talk. I remarked that she did not seem like the same person she was a year ago. She replied, "I'm not, and while I would never wish cancer on anyone, this experience has brought me strength and confidence."

Her cancer experience was not only physical, but spiritual and transformative. She told me that she was divorcing her husband and starting school. Since that time, I have seen transformation in others. She taught me that I will often take care of my patients' emotional needs even more than their medical needs. ❦

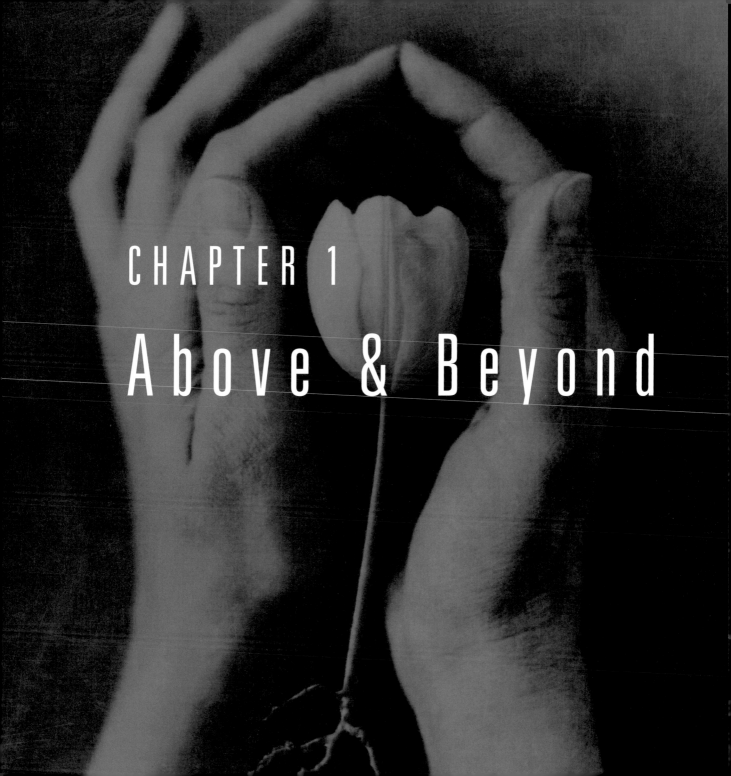

CHAPTER 1
Above & Beyond

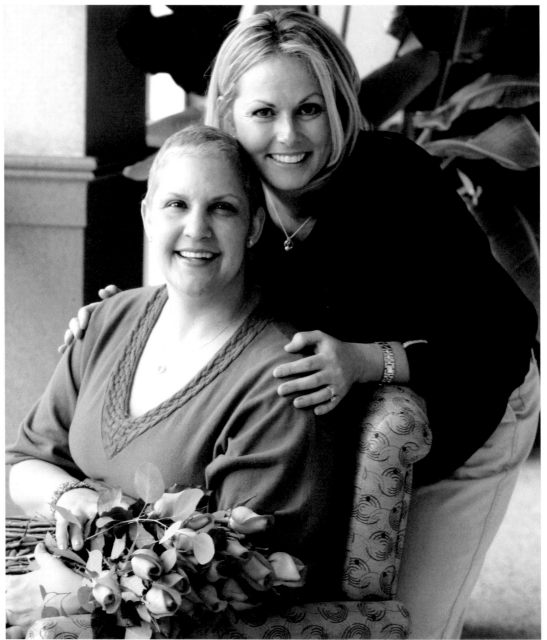

Sharon Britain, RN, CACP, OCN [right] with Karen Mitchell

Not Just a Nurse

SHARON BRITAIN, RN, CACP, OCN [MEMORIAL HEALTH SYSTEM CANCER CENTER IN COLORADO SPRINGS, COLORADO]   WRITTEN BY KAREN MITCHELL

IT IS IMPOSSIBLE to prepare for the diagnosis of breast cancer. Women do things their whole lives to lower their risks, at the same time counting on their genetics to spare them the label of "cancer patient." I have no family history of breast cancer, nursed both my children for three years each, and exercise regularly.

NEVERTHELESS, at the age of 38, with two young children, I had to undergo a biopsy for pain along my rib cage on December 22, 2009. I then had to wait through Christmas for my positive diagnosis. The game plan seemed fairly simple: a mastectomy and reconstructive surgery (which I viewed as a chance to lift my sagging breasts!)—all along hoping I would not be a candidate for chemotherapy. I prayed—along with friends and churches—to avoid chemotherapy. Yet, I clearly recall sitting in my oncologist's office when he recommended chemo. I remember saying to him, tears streaming down my face, "I'm sorry, but could you repeat everything you said since you first suggested chemotherapy 10 minutes ago? I tuned it all out."

Facing chemotherapy is very complex. The word "chemotherapy" seems like a death sentence. Most of the time, those who choose to share a chemo story tell you of a relative who had a horrible experience, fighting unthinkable side effects and, in the end, not surviving. In short, chemo has a terrible reputation.

Enter Sharon Britain. Sharon single-handedly alleviated all of my fears about chemotherapy, gave me strength to face it, and put my life back on track. I doubt Sharon even knows how profoundly she impacts the lives of the patients she serves, as she is as down to earth as a person can be. Talking to Sharon is like chatting with my own sister. She has mastered walking that fine line between lending support and offering privacy.

When I first met Sharon, I was hoping she would tell me that chemotherapy is a breeze, that the stories

I had heard were grossly exaggerated, and that I would not lose my hair, which, for someone who has had long hair her entire life, could be the worst side effect of chemo. She said none of these things. Instead, Sharon spent more than two hours outlining the essentials of chemo. I learned from Sharon that there is comfort and peace in education. A lot of the fear of chemotherapy lies in the unknown. What is it, really? What will it feel like? What are the side effects? And, most important, how badly will it hurt?

That fear of losing my hair? No longer a fear! Sharon understood, helping me try on wigs. She told me funny stories throughout, encouraged me to try wigs I would not normally consider, and made the whole process fun. Seeing how other women dealt with their hair loss took away the shame of losing my hair and the feeling that it is some kind of punishment. My 14-year-old daughter was with me on this visit, and looking at scarves inspired her to make me a head covering as her 4-H level 2 sewing project. Sharon found my daughter a book on how to make a headscarf. She was so excited about making the headscarf that she is also going to make me a matching "chemo shirt," a sleeveless shirt made from a stain-resistant material that is cut to give easy access to the chemo port. As you can see, Sharon brought my daughter onboard, giving her a project—a way she can help me.

TEACHING MOMENT:

She has mastered walking that fine line between lending support and offering privacy.

Sharon has spent a great deal of time answering dozens of my questions about possible side effects of chemotherapy. We have discussed pain management, stress management, family life, sex during chemo, and more. Sharon always has an answer for my questions, often telling me what worked for other women. Again, it is the reassurance from Sharon that thousands of other women have fought the same battle, experienced the same fears, and dealt with the same side effects that gives me the strength to get through this time.

How do I sum up what makes Sharon so special? In a word, Sharon is empowering. She is a straight talker who is also compassionate and gentle. She knows when to talk and when to listen. She knows how to remove the shame from going through chemotherapy. I wish I could have met Sharon under different circumstances because I don't just call her an oncology nurse. I am proud to also call her a friend. ❧

With All Her Heart

PAULA RICHARDSON, BSN, OCN [SAMARITAN AMBULATORY INFUSION CENTER IN CORVALLIS, OREGON]   WRITTEN BY JANET MOSLEY

I WAS DIAGNOSED with stage 3A ovarian cancer in 2001. Two physicians expected the growth to be a common ovarian cyst—go in, clip it out, and get on with life. Not the first misdiagnosis I'm certain—or the last. I was devastated yet determined not to be a cancer patient who hears the "C" word and prepares to die. I would fight. My surgeon recommended Dr. Peter Kenyon as the best oncologist he knew, so I met with Dr. Kenyon and mapped out my future.

DURING MY FIRST VISIT, I was very impressed with his private nurse, Paula Richardson. She was kind, interested, and almost seemed to be one step ahead of the doctor. I bonded with her immediately and her presence visibly calmed me every time I visited the office. She continued to work with Dr. Kenyon through my first round of therapy and the 18-month remission that followed.

When my disease recurred, Paula was the first person I looked for after the doctor's visit, and she held me while I cried and explained many other options available to me in this continuing battle. She refused to leave my side until I was calm and ready to face the world. That day would have been very difficult without her.

As I began my second round of chemo, I learned that Paula had become a chemo nurse in our clinic. This thrilled me since I'd get to "have" her every treatment … if I whined enough! With the exception of a second 18-month remission, I have remained on chemotherapy from then to the present. Paula moved to another chemo infusion center in our town (I followed!) and has been my nurse and my friend throughout this nine-year period.

Please allow me to present a few examples of her loving care.

I reacted to my chemotherapy, after many treatments, by simply sneezing (in a room full of other noisy people). Paula immediately observed from across the room (she was with another patient) and asked why I did that. Within seconds she was across the room, had the drug stopped, was injecting me with antihistamine, taking my blood pressure, and corralling the doctor … all before the other symptoms began to emerge at an alarming rate. She brought me through that episode swiftly and safely with little fuss.

After several years of encouragement, Paula finally convinced me to have a port installed since my hand and arm veins were beginning to disappear. I nervously went to the hospital for the surgery and, of course, there was Paula to sit with me before surgery, be there when I woke, take me to lunch, and see that I got home safely … taking up her entire day off.

I had a debulking surgery recently and, you guessed it, there was Paula, wasting another perfectly good day off to be with me and my family as we waited for my turn in the surgical unit. Her strong, cheerful strength made the whole ordeal much, much easier.

In our area, some new chemo treatments must first be administered in our hospital as a safety precaution. Yes, Paula spent another precious day off with me as I received that five-hour infusion, knitting, talking, laughing, and pretending she wasn't watching every procedure.

TEACHING MOMENT:

She cries when she must, she laughs with the joy of life, and she loves with all her heart.

Paula is a truly remarkable person. It is difficult to fully convey the concern, care, and affection she generates for each and every patient. No matter how busy her day, how short the time, she will hold the hand of a frightened soul and gently explain every nuance of the treatment, what to expect, how the drug will work, the nature of the disease, and not leave until that patient is calmed and more comfortable. If she has to leave for a moment and says she'll be right back, she will. I've seen sorrow in her eyes, yet when she greets a new person, only the pleasure of their meeting shows through. She cries when she must, she laughs with the joy of life, and she loves with all her heart. ❧

A True Friend

KATHY ROTHERING, RN, BSN [UNIVERSITY OF WISCONSIN, HOSPITALS AND CLINICS IN MADISON, WISCONSIN]   WRITTEN BY WENDY WARREN

IN APRIL 2006, during surgery to remove a tumor that was thought to be ovarian cancer, it was discovered that what I indeed had was gastrointestinal stromal tumors, or GIST, a rare cancer. It's nearly impossible to explain what is felt when you wake up from surgery to have a surgeon tell you: "It wasn't what we thought it was. It's GIST; it's rare, widely metastasized, and ah, did we say there's no cure?"

IT WAS THE WORD "incurable" that felt like a knife plunged into my heart. When I asked if I would die, all the surgeon could say was "These are hard times, Wendy." Prior to surgery, I was confident in my ability to be a statistic in the "five-year and beyond" survival category for ovarian cancer patients. Why, with my otherwise great health and fighting spirit, why wouldn't I be?

As the fog cleared over the coming months, I did indeed learn that recently developed "miracle" treatments made my cancer, in many cases, one that you could live many years with before it would progress again. Okay, this I could do! My resolve to fight returned. I quickly realized this was not a fight one embarked on alone. I would need a lot of help and support. It wasn't until 2008 and two years into the fight that I met the most supportive person to date in my four-year journey. Her name is Kathy Rothering, GI nurse coordinator.

Kathy was running the then six-member GI support group that I hesitantly walked into on a Wednesday afternoon. Kathy immediately put me at ease, making me feel welcome. I cried at my very first support group, and she said she "had my back." When I look back now, I ask why I wasn't given information that such a position existed. Prior to meeting Kathy, I felt very alone and without a real connection to anyone at the clinic.

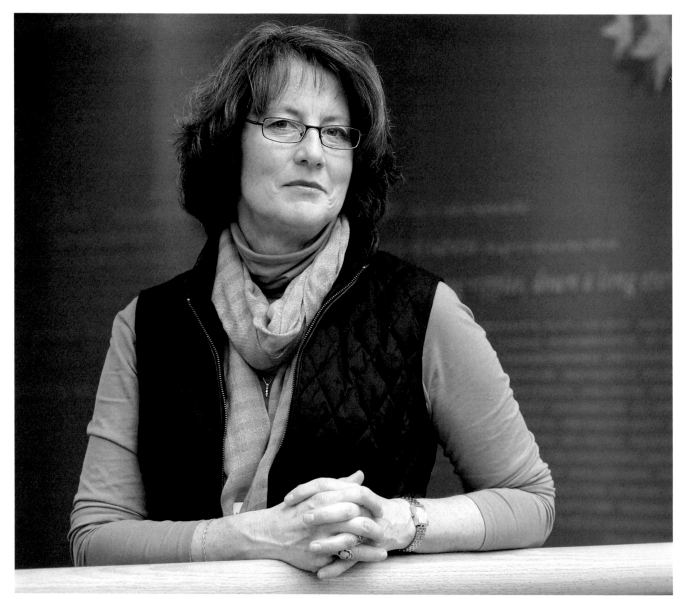

Kathy Rothering, RN, BSN

In 2008, I was struggling to keep up the fight, not just the cancer fight, but the navigating of the "systems" that touch your life because of cancer. What I quickly learned upon meeting Kathy is not just how valuable her services are—after all anyone can hold a title and position. It is how Kathy approaches and carries out her job. Running the support group is a very small but important part of it. As such, she sets up educational speakers, connects members, and participates fully in providing her expertise. Kathy approaches other aspects of her job with efficiency as well as kindness, compassion, and a sense of hopefulness.

Always available by phone or e-mail, Kathy does not hesitate to gather records, juggle appointments to meet my schedule, communicate messages to the doctor, and answer questions about side effects. She makes me feel as if she is my "personal" on-call nurse! In talking to other patients, I know I am not the only person feeling this way. After my second surgery, not only did she come to my room to see me, but when I went home, she spent a great deal of time easing my anxieties regarding symptoms I was having.

TEACHING MOMENT:

She makes me feel as if she is my "personal" on-call nurse!

Our support group has become a fairly close-knit group over time. We have little parties on holidays, hold outings, and have attended a picnic at one member's house. Kathy was there, and it was obvious she genuinely values us all as so much more than just cancer patients.

When we "lost" the member that held the picnic, it was Kathy who broke the news to us as well as organized the card, flowers, and memorial gift we would give as a group. It made a difficult time a tad easier for all.

In addition, Kathy has met me in the waiting room on particularly hard appointment days just to check in and wish me luck. She has interpreted reports for me while holding my hand. And if you have tried to navigate the world of insurance companies, clinics, big hospitals, and employment while living with cancer, you know that everything is difficult times five. But in Kathy, I have found a partner, an ally—a compassionate, true friend to share that difficulty with.

These days my substantial bucket full of issues feels lighter when Kathy, as she so often does, symbolically grabs the other handle and helps me carry it up the proverbial cancer hill. ❧

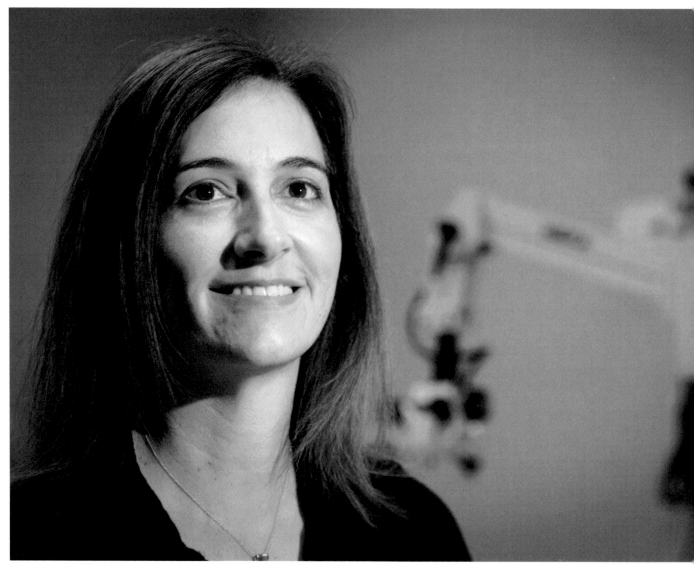

Kim Haley, RN, BSN

Calm Before the Storm

KIM HALEY, RN, BSN [CRESCENT CITY PHYSICIANS IN NEW ORLEANS, LOUISIANA]

WRITTEN BY CHRISTINE DITTMANN

Above &
Beyond

THE CALM before the storm—that lull right before something big happens. For New Orleans, the calm came the last weekend of August 2005—right before Hurricane Katrina came. I thought the calm before "my" storm had come and gone, as I was already undergoing treatment for thyroid cancer when I was diagnosed with stage 4 ovarian cancer, just 18 months after having a complete hysterectomy.

MY GRANDMOTHER DIED of ovarian cancer and my mother of breast cancer. So, at the end of August, my father flew in town to be with me for my first appointment with the gynecologic oncologist, but Hurricane Katrina barreled through, devastating New Orleans and my home. We relocated to New Jersey to stay with family. While there, I received treatment for my thyroid and ovarian cancers, but we missed home and moved back. Just days before our 11th wedding anniversary, I was told the ovarian cancer had returned. I was referred by my gynecologist to gynecologic oncologist Dr. Joan Cheng, which is when I met Kim Haley.

Kim is Dr. Cheng's nurse. She's been a nurse for more than 20 years, and for the last 8 years, she's been working with female cancer patients. Kim was soft-spoken and sweet. And it turns out I would be seeing a lot of Kim in the years to come. Shortly after that first appointment, I underwent my second debulking surgery. Since then, I have had two more surgeries (for a total of four) and a total of 50 chemotherapy treatments. But as hard as the last few years have been, I still feel very blessed by the many wonderful people I've met on this journey, and my oncology nurse Kim is one of those people for so many reasons.

I credit my family, my friends, my faith, my doctors, and very importantly, my relationship with Kim for keeping me alive both physically and emotionally. Kim has been my nurse—and friend—for three years now. She not only cares about my physical well-being, but she cares about my quality of life and my family's well-being too. Kim has helped me and countless others live and deal with a disease and diagnosis that we know could ultimately take our lives.

Gynecologic cancer can be so confusing and so personal, which is why I co-facilitate a gyn-cancer support group at Touro. Our core group of participants have all been touched by Kim's expert and compassionate care. One of the members described how Kim's calm, gracious demeanor gave her peace after first finding out about her cancer diagnosis and being told she'd need chemo. This particular woman is a nurse herself and said Kim is her role model because she's an exemplary clinician with a caring heart.

Kim does everything in her power to make our lives as easy as possible when it comes to our cancer diagnosis and treatment. Several other patients, me included, remember how, during the summer of 2008, Kim made sure each of us had our medical records before we evacuated for Hurricane Gustav so that we could receive our chemo treatments uninterrupted. She even delivered one patient's records to her home to make sure she would have no problems being treated. Here I was facing yet another storm, except this time I had Kim looking out for me. She was my "calm before the storm."

Kim's extraordinary efforts are even noticed by individuals who have never met her in person. My oncology nurse case manager who works with oncology offices daily in several different states said that Kim stands out among the crowd, noting her exceptional understanding of the role a case manager has in regard to the patient's insurance plan. She went on to say that Kim is always willing to discuss the patient's plan of care in addressing the specific needs of her patients.

Typically, you experience the calm before the storm, the storm passes, and then you do your best to go back to normal. I realize my storm may never pass, and my life may never be "normal" again. But when my time comes when I won't want to take treatment anymore, I already know Kim will support me in that decision—and that is something very important to me. I will forever be grateful to Kim for all that she's done for me and so will the many other people whose lives she has touched as an extraordinary oncology nurse. ❧

Christine Dittman passed away in September 2010. We are proud to honor her memory.

Dancing with Bonnie

BONNIE STRUDAS, RN, BSN, OCN [MASSACHUSETTS GENERAL HOSPITAL IN BOSTON, MASSACHUSETTS]

WRITTEN BY KAREN LIST

MY DAUGHTER EMILY danced up the driveway on that soft spring day in May 2008, her ballerina's body lifting effortlessly off the gravel as she reached her right arm toward the sky. I watched her and wondered: How can she be dancing when she's just been told she has an egg-size tumor under her left eye?

Above & Beyond

I KNOW NOW that Emily, my then 24-year-old dancer, singer, and actor, home from working in the London Theater, was dancing to gather her courage for what lay ahead. What we couldn't know that day was that her chemo nurse, Bonnie Strudas, would be dancing right along with her.

Bonnie was Emily's infusion nurse after she was diagnosed with a rare pediatric sarcoma. Ten months of difficult treatment caused Emily to lose her hair, 30 pounds from her dancer's frame and, at times, her ability to walk and talk. It was a long haul for a young woman whose life had been interrupted. But Bonnie, right from the start, made Emily, her dad, her little sister, and me feel that we were on a quest for a cure along with her. And if you're on that quest, believe me, Bonnie is the nurse with whom you want to be dancing.

The best reason to have Bonnie as our partner was her extraordinary professionalism, experience, and commitment that allowed Emily and all of us to trust her fully. Not even Emily was dancing the day we first walked into the infusion center. We had little idea about what would happen, how Emily would feel, or whose hands our precious daughter would be in. From the first day, we were grateful they were Bonnie's hands.

Without fail, she explained to Emily every step in the process, making her a full partner in her own treatment. And then she carried out that treatment with great discipline and attention to every detail. Even when I thought Emily might be too tired or too ill to care, Bonnie stroked her head and gently told her what was

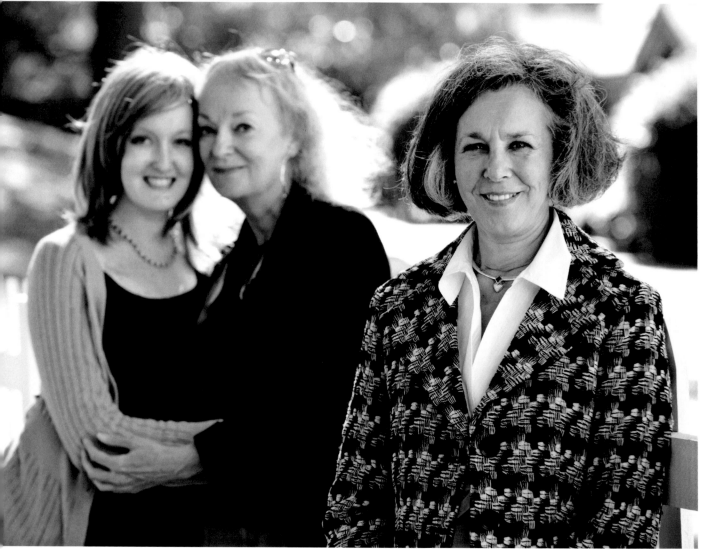

Bonnie Strudas, RN, BSN, OCN [front] with Karen [back right] and Emily List

about to happen, and Emily always responded.

Though the infusion unit was perpetually hopping, Bonnie always took the time to answer questions. If I needed her advice, then and now, she always responded. A year after chemo ended, I find myself saying to doctors, "I'll ask Bonnie." I do, and she answers. Emily and I feel as if she's our partner for life.

Bonnie's vast knowledge is paired with caring and compassion. She always gave Emily the opportunity to talk about her life outside the hospital, treating her like the person she is—not the disease she had. For weeks, Emily hadn't been able to talk—let alone sing—because of radiation burn, but once her voice was back, we sang 1960s songs with Lori, the music therapist, with Bonnie popping in and out of the room to sing with us.

TEACHING MOMENT:

She always gave Emily the opportunity to talk about her life outside the hospital, treating her like the person she is—not the disease she had.

Bonnie was always amazing, but especially the week after Emily's 25th birthday. Emily was to have a chemo treatment on her birthday, but an ice storm kept us home. When we came in, Bonnie had a special birthday hat for Emily, flowers, a gift, and a huge cake. The fact that Bonnie had planned such a party once is unbelievable: but twice?

On Emily's last day of treatment, Lori came by for a farewell song fest. One of the songs Emily chose was "My Guy," and since it obviously was dedicated to her doctor, David Harmon, Bonnie called him. Within minutes, Emily—in bed—our entire family, Lori, Bonnie, several other nurses, and Dr. Harmon himself were all dancing around her room. We will never, ever forget that day.

When Emily was back to have a benign spot removed from her lung, she was hurting and sad when we heard: "I've been looking everywhere for you!" Emily sat up with a shot, smiling for the first time in days. "Bonnie!" she said. Simply put, seeing Bonnie made Emily better. This was the final proof, if any were needed, of the kind of oncology nurse she is and why, among the many bright lights in this field, Bonnie is neon. And she can dance too. ❧

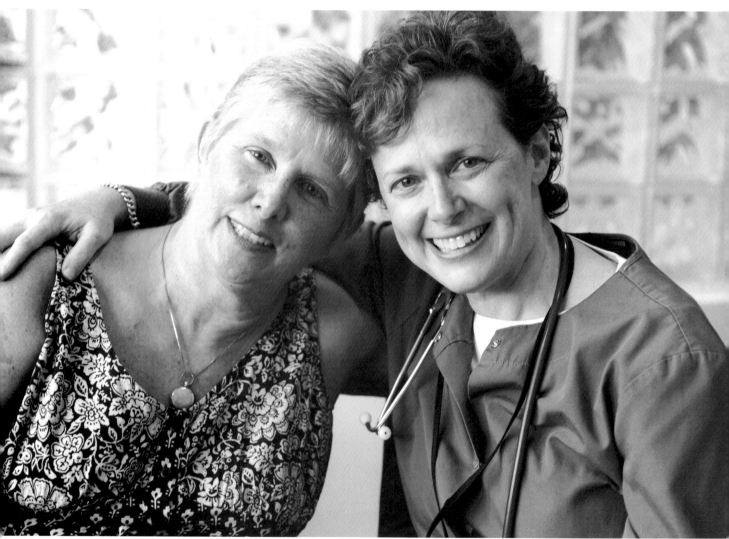

Michelle Beil, RN, BS, OCN [right] with Louise Kuklis

Whirling Dervish

MICHELLE BEIL, RN, BS, OCN [WHITE PLAINS HOSPITAL LOWENTHAL INFUSION CENTER IN WHITE PLAINS, NEW YORK]   WRITTEN BY LOUISE KUKLIS

AS YOU OPEN the door to the infusion center, you would think that you were entering a neighborhood party. You hear laughter and stories and offers of refreshments. This upbeat environment is the home of the "whirling dervish" of oncology nurses, Michelle Beil.

SHE WELCOMES ALL with a hug and specific question about something important in their lives, which of course she has remembered from the patient's last visit. Michelle has made me a cancer survivor.

I was first diagnosed with stage 2 colon cancer back in 2007. I was a nervous wreck the first time I showed up for my chemotherapy, and I would have to make it through 12 treatments! As a teacher and a mother, I worried about leaving my students and not being ready for my son's wedding that summer. Michelle met me at the door and made me feel like a queen as she guided me to my throne (infusion chair).

Michelle was quite the role model for all the patients at the infusion center because she herself was completing treatments for breast cancer. She wore a colorful scarf to cover the evidence of her chemotherapy and radiation. Nevertheless she was full of energy and optimism. Yet she was also willing to share her own worries about facing cancer and its impact on her family, which comforted the rest of us with similar concerns.

With great confidence she accessed my port that first day and explained the effects of the chemotherapy. She also helped to set up my port-a-pump so that I would only have one day at the infusion center and the rest of the treatment could be done at home. She encouraged me to walk and to enjoy my time at home. She also called to make sure all was going well. Now I knew I could get through the 12 treatments!

Around treatment seven, my son announced that he wanted to postpone his wedding because of his worries that I would be too sick to enjoy the wedding. Michelle and her team of nurses assured him and his fiancée that they should continue with their summer wedding plans. After treatment 12, Michelle and her fellow nurses donned their cheerleading outfits to celebrate the end of my treatment (a ritual performed for all patients at treatment's end). Then on July 29, I witnessed my son's wedding with tears of joy.

Michelle followed me through the next two years when I had my port cleaned. She would hug me every time and always ask about my family and students. In May 2009, my port was removed. Then my first grandson was born in late June. Michelle celebrated these milestones with me, only to cry with me when two months later CT scans determined that my colon cancer had spread to my lungs. I was now facing stage 4 colon cancer; now I would really need my "whirling dervish!"

At first I was put into the hospital to get my chemotherapy treatments. Michelle and the infusion center administrator found a way to get me home. Michelle and her team went to work to find me a port-a-pump.

Just before Christmas, when my grandson and daughter were visiting, I received my first full chemotherapy treatment in the infusion center, going home with the port-a-pump. Now I was able to witness my grandson's first Christmas.

TEACHING MOMENT:

She was also willing to share her own worries about facing cancer and its impact on her family, which comforted the rest of us with similar concerns.

The amazing thing is that, what Michelle has done for me, she would do for any patient at the infusion center. She can charm the most recalcitrant patient to stay to finish their treatment or to smile. She can speedily access a difficult vein and then race across the room to assist a patient who is feeling nauseous. I have watched her manage a fire alarm evacuation in the midst of winter with so many patients that they were sitting in chairs in the hall.

Michelle has watched over me as I have gone through almost seven months of chemotherapy now. She got me more recovery time from the drugs, which has added to my quality of life. My admiration for Michelle has grown exponentially as I have been in her care. ❧

My Lifeline

VADIM BORCHENKO, RN, OCN [TOWER HEMATOLOGY AND ONCOLOGY IN BEVERLY HILLS, CALIFORNIA]   WRITTEN BY BRENDA DOROGI

ON JANUARY 7, 2008, I received the devastating news that I had stage 3 rectal cancer. In the months that followed, I went through surgery, radiation, and chemotherapy. By October, my scan showed "no evidence of disease," and I went back to what had been my normal life.

THEN, JUST SIX MONTHS LATER, I received the even more devastating news that the cancer had metastasized to my lungs. However, the tumors were too small to treat, and the waiting game began. Finally, in October 2009, the tumors had doubled in size, and I entered chemotherapy again. That is when the real trouble began. And it is also when I met Vadim Borchenko, the extraordinary oncology nurse who would literally save my life and then go on to become the lifeline to bring me through months of grueling chemo.

I am fortunate to be a patient in one of the largest, busiest, and most well-respected cancer centers in Los Angeles. Due to the dynamics of such a busy center, nurses are frequently called on to assist each other, sometimes at a moment's notice. No matter how busy they are, they are always ready to lend a hand.

Vadim excels in this environment. He has the unique ability to manage the multiple demands on his time and the interruptions that inevitably arise and still give full attention to his patients. I have never known Vadim to fail to follow through—whether it is providing nursing care and support throughout an individual chemo session for one of his patients or lending assistance to a fellow nurse.

When Vadim does my chemo treatment, he always gives that little extra level of care, from painlessly accessing my port to miraculously finding a "special" kind of tape when he saw that my skin would not tolerate even paper tape and a quick smile that says "You can do it. I am here for you."

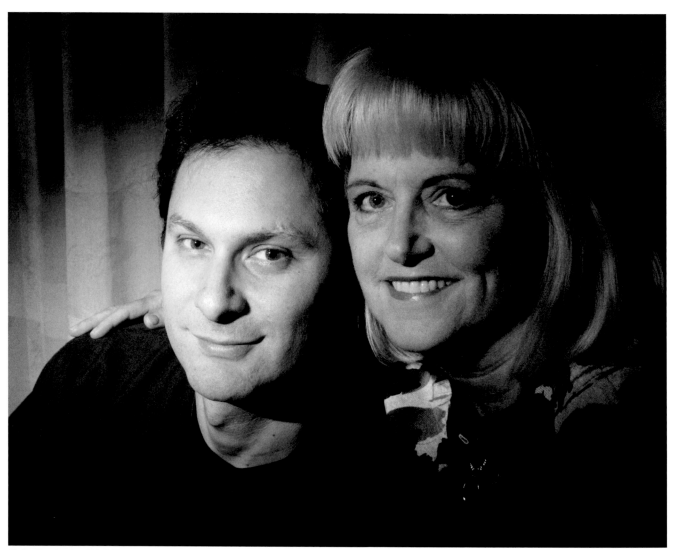

Vadim Borchenko, RN, OCN, with Brenda Dorogi

But that is not all. Quite simply, Vadim saved my life.

I am not an easy patient to care for. My system does not metabolize normally, and I have had severe allergic reactions to many antibiotics, pain killers, and other medications throughout my life. Needless to say, chemo tops them all! I need home nursing care for several days after each chemo session. Fortunately for me, Vadim also does home care, and he is my home nurse.

Initially, I was placed on a standard chemotherapy regimen for rectal cancer. Each treatment became progressively worse. Vadim reacted quickly and knowledgeably, working with the rest of my medical team to add pre- and post-treatment medications to alleviate the nausea and other symptoms. All along the way, he provided emotional support as well, encouraging me to tackle one day at a time, especially when it seemed like it would never end and I wanted to give up and abandon the treatment altogether.

After the third chemo session, I sensed that something was very wrong but was too sick and weak to talk. Vadim took one look at me and saw it right away. Instead of starting the usual treatment, he immediately drew blood for testing and instructed my husband to drive me to the oncology center right away.

In the meantime, he alerted the staff, and by the time we got there, everything was ready for us. Since the test results showed I was having a severe toxic reaction, Vadim had already notified the nurse practitioner and my oncologist, and a treatment plan was developed. Thanks to Vadim's professional instinct, his expertise in assessing my condition, and his prompt action, I am alive today.

Vadim is also my ongoing lifeline. I am still in treatment and still need home health care. Vadim is alert to exactly what the status of my recovery is each day. He is ready to respond with the right medication, if needed, and also with the right words to get me through it. He reminds me that it doesn't last forever. My chemo treatments are on Monday. When I start getting really sick by Wednesday, he promises that I will "feel much better on Sunday." Again, he is always right, and by Sunday I start to feel human again.

Vadim demonstrates the true meaning of nursing care. He adds the personal touch, sensing and empathizing with my pain, sharing my relief when it is over. By believing in me, he gives me the courage to do it all over again. Vadim has helped me realize that my life is not defined by either the cancer or the chemo. Because he sees me as a person instead of just a patient, I can see myself that way, too. ❦

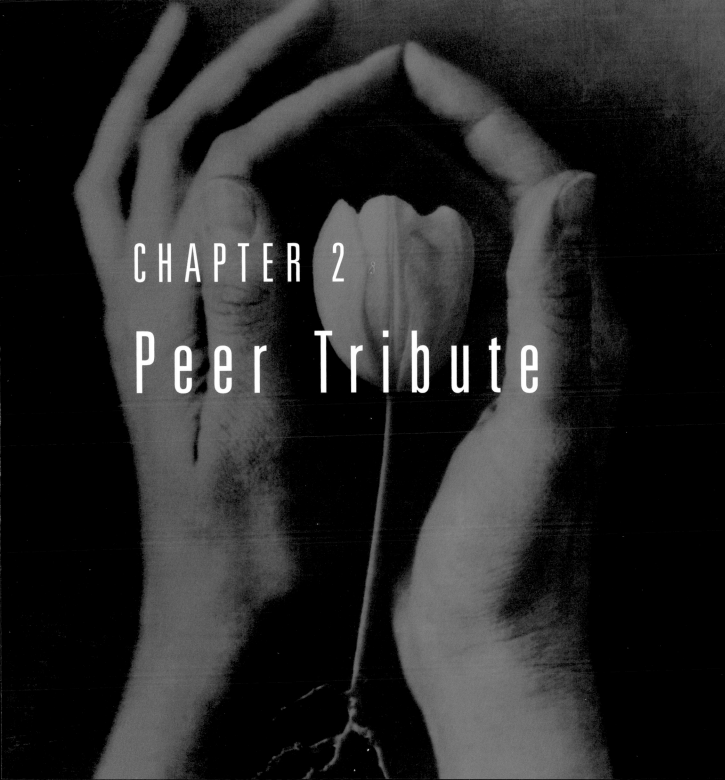

CHAPTER 2
Peer Tribute

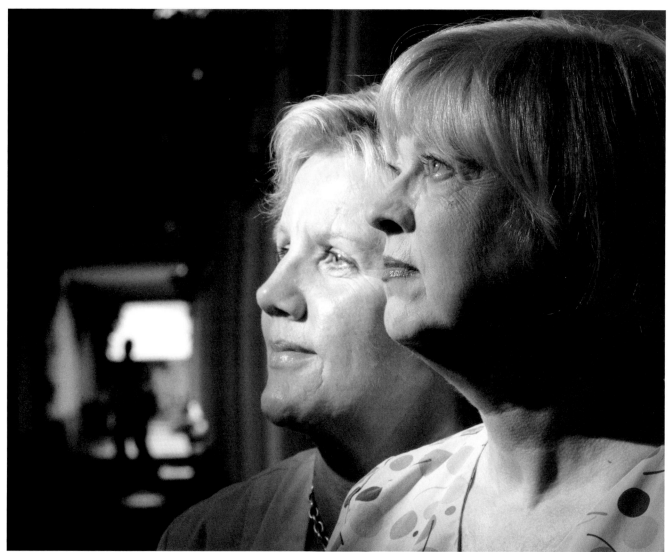

Sharon Thacker, RN [front] with Ann Brady, RN

Priceless

SHARON THACKER, RN [HUNTINGTON MEMORIAL HOSPITAL IN PASADENA, CALIFORNIA]

WRITTEN BY ANN BRADY, RN

Peer Tribute

SHARON CRIED WHEN I said, "thank you." It reminded me of how easy it was to forget the common courtesy of thanking someone for a job well-done. In oncology care, a job well-done often ends with the patient dying. I thanked her because I'd seen the difference she made in the last hours of Mary's life. Sharon allowed Mary the dignity of delaying the start of her pain medication until she had a chance to say goodbye in the way she wanted to.

IN ONCOLOGY, the goodbyes are important. I can't think of any cancer diagnosis that is fair, yet some seem particularly unfair. A rapidly growing pancreatic cancer put Mary into our care. A greedy, painful lesion had multiplied like a parasite and was poised to destroy her. From diagnosis to death was a short three weeks—not enough time for anyone to adjust. Mary saw the writing on the wall before the rest of her family did. They wanted a cure, needed a possibility of treatment to help them make sense of her senseless disease.

Mary was the same age as Sharon. She had a beautiful daughter, nearly the same age as Sharon's daughter. One afternoon Sharon overheard Mary say to her daughter, "Honey, you're going to be okay." A mother comforting her daughter over an upcoming loss. When Sharon told me the story she added, "Why her and not me?" Then she said, almost in a whisper, "What would I tell my daughter if I were dying of cancer?" It's a question we all struggle with. Why do some people get cancer? I watched Sharon the next day as she spoke to the daughter outside Mary's room. Explaining what to expect of the disease, providing support, and teaching.

Sharon stood close, one hand on the daughter's arm. I knew she had figured out what to say.

Sharon mentored me when I was a newly graduated nurse. I've watched her teach other new nurses and heard her instructing and educating patients about cancer. She has a knack for finding strategies to improve the patient's experience. She knows how to comfort at the right time and to step back at other times. She knows that each patient's illness is unique, and she remembers that as she cares for them. She has been a nurse long enough not to let her knowledge of the outcome alter her care. Discretion can take years to perfect.

Oncology care extracts a high price from the nurse. To balance the emotional toll, it helps to find meaning in the experience, though sometimes it is not easily found. Sharon found that delicate balance. She worried about Mary. "She's weak yet so determined. I wish there were something more I could do for her." If it was up to Sharon, she would have given Mary more pain medication to make her comfortable, but Mary explained why she wanted to wait—that she wanted to say goodbye clear headed. Sometimes as nurses, we want to override the patient's wishes because it would be easier. After all, we've seen it before; we know what comes next. But Sharon listened to Mary and let her decide.

While they waited for the brother to get there, Sharon explained how a little medication could decrease Mary's pain without altering her alert state—how she could calibrate the meds to achieve both results. Then Mary would be comfortable enough to say goodbye. They agreed on a little medication while she waited; then once the brother arrived, Sharon would start the drip. It wasn't an easy conversation to have. It took compassion on Sharon's part to honor that the experience was unique to Mary, to guide her without pushing.

On her last day, Mary's husband and daughter sat on each side of her. When her brother arrived, there were tears of relief and sadness. Peace. He took her hand and nodded. No words were necessary. Sharon waited a few minutes before starting the narcotics. Mary nodded to Sharon, mouthed the words, "thank you." Later Sharon said, "You could feel the love in that room." It only took an hour. Mary had held on, but with her goodbyes done, she accepted the unacceptable. Sharon helped her achieve her goal, a priceless instance of excellent nursing care. I thanked her because she did a good job. But I also thanked her because the way she cared for Mary showed all of us—nurses and patients and their families—what a difference great nursing care makes. Sharon makes me want to be a better nurse. ❦

A Bright Spirit

EMILY FAGAN, RN [MONROE CARELL JR. CHILDREN'S HOSPITAL AT VANDERBILT IN NASHVILLE, TENNESSEE]

WRITTEN BY BY CAROLINE HALE

Peer Tribute

THERE IS *NO* substitute for a high-quality care provider—especially in the childhood cancer world. In 2000 when I was diagnosed with cancer at 13, this simple fact became very evident to my family and me. Because cancer entered my life at the onset of my adolescent years—and the majority of patients being treated were significantly younger than I—the many days I spent in clinic were filled with conversation with parents of children with cancer and with nurses. I am now eight years post-treatment, and still, my heart swells every time I think of my oncology nurses. My family and I love each nurse beyond measure, but one stands out in my mind without question—Emily Fagan.

IF YOU'VE MET a most compassionate person who can bring a smile to the face of everyone she encounters and never, ever allows her hard day to reflect in her actions, then you've likely met a person who embodies *no more than half of* Emily's caring nature. I understand the power a single example can have, but I believe that the continual bright spirit of a care provider handily outweighs the impact of one story.

During every single day of my two-year treatment, Emily let her bright spirit shine. She gave, and continues to gives, all of herself to the children and families she serves. For a teenage girl with cancer, the occurrence of a smile seems somewhat far-fetched. I am *not* over-exaggerating when I state that, amid the terrible

47

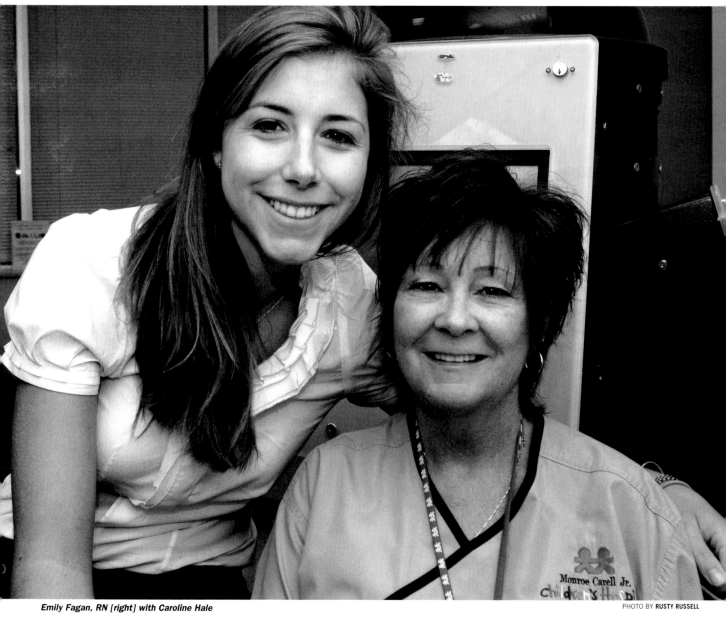

Emily Fagan, RN [right] with Caroline Hale

side effects that accompany chemotherapy treatment and the isolation from my friends, Emily made me smile every time I was around her. Because a smile will instantaneously lift one's mood, when Emily was around, my day immediately became better.

Emily continually went beyond the call of duty to help me. Certain drugs, when given in high doses, as most cancer survivors know, will dramatically increase a person's appetite. For a period of time I was taking a medication that would result in crazy hunger pains. Countless times, Emily would search all the cabinets for any remaining bags of my favorite chips.

I beat cancer, and I'm told that I'm strong. But, I wholly believe that "strong" does not begin to describe the abilities of pediatric oncology nurses, especially Emily. It is inconceivable for me to understand how Emily, amid all of the sadness in a pediatric oncology outpatient clinic, is able to put on a smile and provide a loving and caring touch, every minute of every day.

TEACHING MOMENT:

Because a smile will instantaneously lift one's mood, when Emily was around, my day immediately became better.

Peer Tribute

I stated that there is no substitute for a high-quality care provider, and "high-quality" in my understanding is defined by Emily. My love for Emily, and the other oncology faculty and staff who cared for me, is so great that my only job since high school has been working at the Children's Hospital. I graduated from college in May 2009, and immediately I began year one of a career at Children's. While I'm only 22 years old, I can safely say that there are few greater joys in life than walking the halls of the hospital and seeing members of my care team every day. ❧

A Place of Life

APRIL DAVIS, RN, OCN [CANCER CENTER OF THE CAROLINAS IN GREENVILLE, SOUTH CAROLINA]

WRITTEN BY M. JEAN LILLEY, RN, BSN

IT HAS BEEN less than two years since I found out I had a very aggressive form of breast cancer, and a year since my doctor happily informed me I had a miraculous, complete clinical remission of the cancer! Being a registered nurse for more than 30 years, I have not forgotten the "beyond the call of duty" professionalism from various health care personnel. I cannot honor each one but will always remember how each helped me in their own special way along my life journey.

SOME EARLY MEMORIES that "touched my heart" were the genuine requested hug that was returned from my nurse practitioner as I began the journey of testing the "lump," and the wonderful requested prayer from the breast navigator as she knelt in front of my husband and me on the day of the "official diagnosis." From doctors to technicians, there was no lack of caring persons. Through all the days of uncertainty and confusion, the exceptional quality of care from health care workers, coupled with prayers, faith, and hope, all helped soften the harshness of the days that would follow.

The first memory of my special nurse was through the vital role of a co-worker. Not everyone is fortunate to have a co-worker who is employed as one of the research nurses at your oncology doctor's office. Believing nothing happens by chance, I will always be grateful for my friend's help in navigating me through the difficult initial journey of breast cancer treatment by taking me on a short tour of the chemotherapy room. Thinking back on her many acts of kindness, I will always believe the most important one was taking time to introduce me to my future chemotherapy nurse, April Davis. April's smile, kindness, and attentiveness during this brief meeting on a busy day built a trust that would be tested when my chemo would start just a few weeks later.

April's dedication and personalized attention helped calm my fears on that initial day of chemo in which I received three chemo agents with other meds. Those meds continued as a part of my personal treatment every three weeks and lasted for more than three months. April not only explained each med and possible side effects but also sat by my chair to monitor for adverse reactions. Although close monitoring is required protocol for administering chemotherapeutic agents to new patients, April's reassuring presence is what I remembered as I came for each treatment. Her careful attention to my needs never wavered, no matter how busy the day.

The chemo room was made as "homey" as possible, but these comforts would have made little difference without the exceptional care by April and the entire chemo staff. Being present for more than three hours for treatments, I had plenty of time to watch the care that was given to each patient. As I observed patients reading books or magazines, listening through CD headsets, or sleeping with pillows and blankets tucked around them, the best part was watching April make each patient feel special, as if they were her only patient. Phone calls from patients received the same individualized attention. My husband was with me for each treatment, and April extended her compassionate care to him also.

Sometimes a first impression can be deceiving, but April's sweet disposition, kindness, cheerfulness, and loving care remained the same from the first meeting. Her knowledgeable care and acts of compassion kept me returning to those hanging bags of fluids without apprehension. I'm sure April's obvious love of oncology nursing helped me see the chemo room as a place of life, rather than a place of avoiding death.

Because ministry has always been so important in what I do as a nurse, I am thankful for the lasting impressions of comfort and care that April has left on my life. Always while resting in the blue rocker recliner, I felt safe and secure under April's watchful eye. I will cherish those memories in the chemo room as part of the incredible cancer journey that challenged my spiritual beliefs and forced me to grow in ways that would never have been possible. I am thankful April was a part of that life-altering experience that causes me to continue to reach out to other cancer patients through my nursing and sharing my personal story in hopes of easing their burdens along the difficult journey of breast cancer. ❧

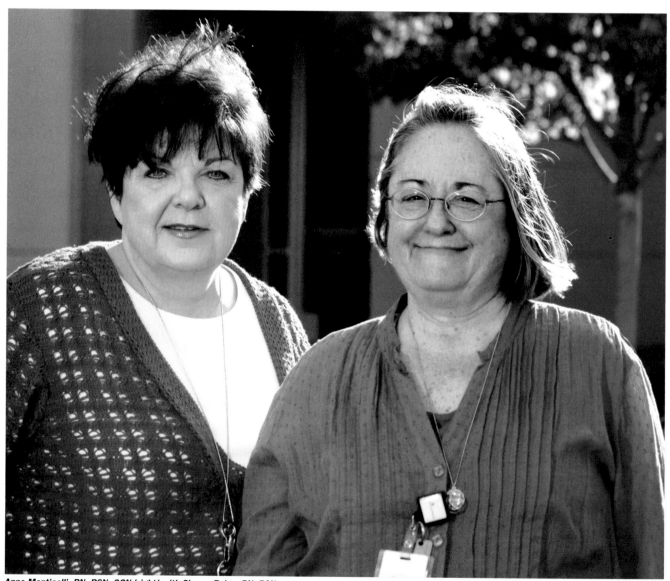

Anne Monticelli, RN, BSN, OCN [right] with Sharon Baker, RN, BSN

Daily Inspiration

ANNE MONTICELLI, RN, BSN, OCN [LASH GROUP, AMERISOURCEBERGEN SPECIALTY GROUP IN FRISCO, TEXAS]   WRITTEN BY SHARON BAKER, RN, BSN

WHEN I WAS a young child, my mother worked at a world-renowned cancer hospital on the pediatric floor. I grew up with stories from there, and few had happy endings. When I reached my preteens, I donated all of my dolls to that floor. One in particular I chose for a special little girl from another country who had acute leukemia. I could only imagine how scared she was, not speaking the language and having such an awful disease. I hoped the doll would bring her some comfort during her battle. It was then that leukemia became one of the two biggest fears in my life.

Peer Tribute

I GREW UP to become a nurse and started my career in pediatric intensive care. After that, I worked in adult cardiology research before going back into a pediatric hospital in management. For 22 years, I avoided direct contact with oncology, as though cancer would not notice me if I didn't make contact with it.

Then several things happened. I went to a new internal medicine doctor who wanted to do a basic physical with labs. When my platelet count came back a little low, I blew it off—but he didn't. I was a healthy mom with an 8-year-old daughter! Repeat labs continued to show small decreases until I became impatient and convinced it was lab error. I had a CBC through employee health. To my horror, I had acute myeloid leukemia (AML) blast cells on a peripheral smear. No taser could have stunned me more! My fear was suffocating. I remember little else until I was in the hospital having my central line placed. And then I met Anne.

Anne talked to me, telling me what was happening, when it would happen, what to expect. Day in and day out, Anne calmed me, educated me, guided me, encouraged me, and reassured me. She anticipated setbacks and side effects. My 80-year-old mother stayed with me during the day most of the time, but if I knew Anne was on, my mom could go home and rest. I was convinced I would survive the shift if Anne was there. In fact, if Anne was there, I could rest too.

I completed induction therapy and two rounds of consolidation. Each time I went into the hospital, my security depended on Anne being there. At one point, I developed a fungal infection, and the medical photographer took pictures of my face. Anne covered the mirror and convinced me I did not want to look. Another time, Anne told me I should not try to get out of bed. What do they say about nurses being patients? I scooted out the bottom of the bed, only to find myself laid out on the floor. Anne was standing over me, shaking her index finger and scolding me. I almost laughed. During transfusions, when I would flip around like a fish, Anne was there in a flash, pushing drugs to make it stop. One night, when my platelets were really low, Anne assured me that the single-donor platelets that were coming would sustain me, and I felt hope.

I was a better nurse because I learned directly from the hands of the best.

During that most horrible time of my life, Anne showed me what it means to be a really great nurse. When I went back to work, a doctor asked me if I was a better nurse after having gone through AML. I told him, no, I was a better nurse because I learned directly from the hands of the best. I truly believe I am alive today because I had the best nurse ever.

As if to complete the circle, I now work with oncology patients, and I never lose focus. Like most cancer survivors, I want to give back 100 percent. I want to be as good for my patients as Anne was for me. The icing on my cake is that I still have Anne with me, but now she is my peer. We work together, and she inspires me every day! ❧

Grace Under Pressure

JOANNA LUPARDUS, RN, BSN, OCN [MARIETTA MEMORIAL HOSPITAL IN MARIETTA, OHIO]

WRITTEN BY TRICIA BECKER, RN, OCN

WHEN I WAS a new nurse on the medical-surgical unit at our small hospital, I was afraid of the patients with cancer. I was afraid that I would do something wrong to cause the patient more pain, more anxiety than they already were experiencing. The I.V. therapy team took care of delivering the chemotherapy drugs.

THERE WAS ONE I.V. therapy nurse in particular who knew those oncology patients inside and out. Joanna knew what medications they were getting and why, what side effects to watch for, and what to do to make the patients more comfortable. The hospital had opened an outpatient oncology clinic, and Joanna was working most of her hours there but still covered some of the I.V. therapy hours on the floors.

As I became more experienced, I became more comfortable caring for our inpatient oncology patients, but caring for them full-time was the furthest thing from my mind. There was a job posting for the outpatient clinic, and I remember thinking, "Who could do that job day in and day out? Certainly not me." But God began working on me and telling me, "Yes, you can."

After applying for a job twice, I was hired. Joanna quickly became the nurse I looked up to the most. I was taught from the beginning to treat everyone as I would want to be treated because all it takes is that one X-ray or test, and it is us sitting in that treatment chair.

She has a calming influence in any situation. If a patient is having a reaction, she gives the drugs to counteract it and talks the patient through it with a reassuring smile. When patients are unsure about their prognosis, she sits next to them, looks them in the eye, and helps them "prepare for the worst, but hope for the best." When the doctors are upset and yelling about their patient schedule being behind, she calmly replies,

"Let's sit down at the end of the day and see what we could do differently."

It was Joanna's dream that we could offer our patients the opportunity to participate in clinical trials. The closest options for our patients were to travel to Columbus, Cleveland, or Pittsburgh—away from their homes and families. So Joanna did some research and lots of convincing that this was a desperately needed service for the people in our area.

Marietta Memorial Hospital, Strecker Cancer Center entered into an agreement with the Columbus CCOP in 2002. She struggled to get the program up and running with our first patients while maintaining her regular workload. Our clinical trials program has grown to the point that we needed a full-time nurse to take care of it. I gladly accepted that role two years ago. I have learned so much from Joanna in the time I have worked in the cancer center, not only about oncology, but about the kind of person I want to be—to have grace under pressure. ❧

TEACHING MOMENT:

She has a calming influence in any situation. If a patient is having a reaction, she gives the drugs to counteract it and talks the patient through it with a reassuring smile.

Compassion Personified

LEEANNE FENNEY, RN [BAYSTATE MEDICAL CENTER/SPRINGFIELD 3 ONCOLOGY IN SPRINGFIELD, MASSACHUSETTS]   WRITTEN BY PAM FISK, RN, CHPN

LEEANNE RADIATES compassion. When a person calls to mind the image of an oncology nurse, Leeanne would be the nurse who exhibits all the characteristics of that consummate oncology caregiver. There are so many ways that she contributes to the well-being of our patients and also to the quality care given by our nurses through role-modeling and sharing oncology knowledge and expertise.

SPRINGFIELD 3 Oncology at Baystate Medical Center is a 23-bed, very busy inpatient oncology unit with an extraordinary staff. We care for many patients with leukemia and lymphoma from the ages of 18 and older. This means that we develop relationships with both the patients and their families and see them often from initial diagnosis through whatever treatments and outcomes their diagnosis leads them—including end-of-life decisions and care.

One patient, of many, who comes to mind as an example of the care Leeanne provides was Stephanie. Stephanie was 19 years old, transferred from a small local hospital with acute abdominal and back pain. Her diagnosis was B-cell lymphoma. She came with her mother and many friends and was frightened and desperate for information. Leeanne immediately set to making both Stephanie and her mother more comfortable. She kept them informed and offered many hugs and words of comfort. Their bond was tight and Leeanne cared for Stephanie through diagnosis, chemotherapy, radiation, continued progression of disease, and finally the conversation that all were dreading. Stephanie's mother really needed Leeanne's support and comfort, and no matter how busy she was, Leeanne was there for them. She remains in touch with that family. Stephanie has been gone for two years.

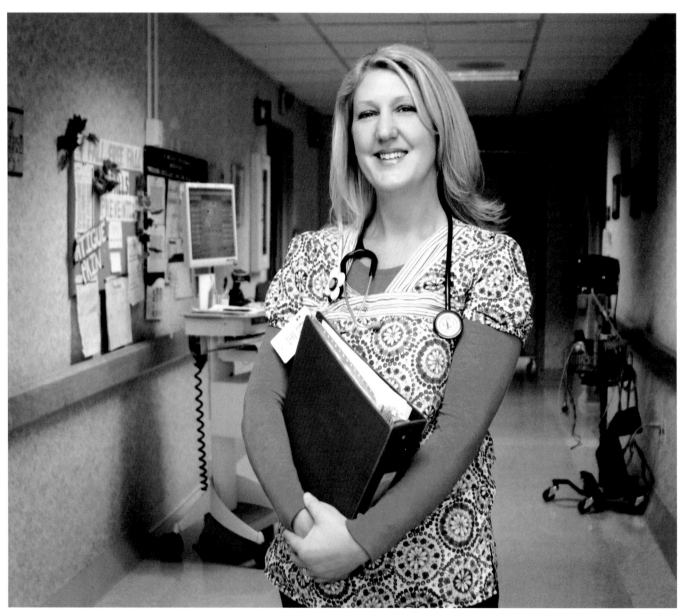

Leeanne Fenney, RN

There are so many examples of Leeanne's care that it is hard to choose which ones to share. She works to pull together an often fragmented approach to care and ensures that the patient remains the focus. She educates, informs, and provides support and impeccable care to her patients.

Springfield 3 Oncology is not the only unit to benefit from Leeanne's expertise. One of the nurses on another unit had a patient with a new diagnosis and felt she needed a consult with an oncology nurse to better serve her patient. She came on to our unit and was met by Leeanne. Leeanne not only shared clinical information with the nurse but then went to the patient's bedside to offer support to him and his wife. The nurse was so moved by Leeanne's support, both to her and the patient, that she shared it in a clinical narrative that will be available to all nurses in our institution to read.

Leeanne is herself a cancer survivor. I've been told that, through it all, she continued her work and never stopped giving of herself. I can only imagine that this experience has brought a new dimension to her level of compassion and empathy. She only shares this information with patients when she feels it would be beneficial. Otherwise, it is rarely mentioned.

What is most special about Leeanne is her ability to make patients feel that she is with them, wholly and completely. I have watched her make patients and families feel that they are the most important people in the world at that moment. She never rushes, never makes her patients feel she has other tasks to be done—no matter what her assignment is or what other pressures exist; and we all know they exist on a busy oncology unit. It is not uncommon to find Leeanne sitting on a patient's bed, holding their hand or tucked in a corner quietly explaining a situation or comforting a family member. When you watch Leeanne physically care for a patient, it is as though she is caring for her own family member. She attends to that patient with gentleness, sincerity, and always the utmost respect. She has amazing conversations with patients; she's comfortable approaching the subject of end of life with families. She is respected by her co-workers and physicians, social workers and case managers, and especially patients and their families.

Leeanne has always provided superior care with compassion and respect throughout her career. It is an honor to work with her. ❧

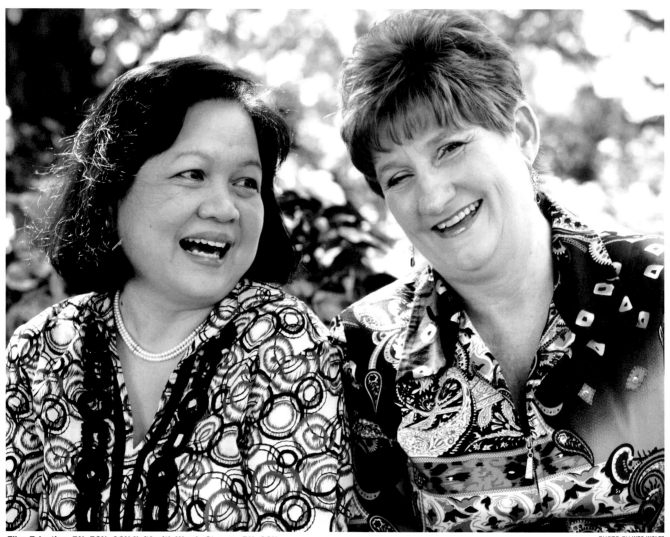

Ellen Tolentino, RN, BSN, OCN [left] with Wanda Strange, RN, OCN

On the Front Line

ELLEN TOLENTINO, RN, BSN, OCN [BAYLOR A. CHARLES SAMMONS CANCER CENTER IN DALLAS, TEXAS]

WRITTEN BY WANDA STRANGE, RN, OCN

OVER THE PAST decade, it has been my privilege to work alongside some of the finest nurses in the profession. For these nurses, oncology is much more than a career: it is a calling. To choose one of these extraordinary nurses is difficult, as each one is special to me. Today, I choose to honor Ellen Tolentino, who stands out as an extraordinary nurse among these amazing caregivers.

Peer Tribute

I HAD BEEN working as an oncology nurse insurance coordinator for about one year when I completed the course work to transition from licensed vocational nurse to registered nurse. My fellow nurses became cheerleaders, always quick with words of encouragement. My first close encounter with Ellen was during this time. I had limited experience with I.V. access and infusion pumps and was very nervous about that portion of my exam. As the time neared for my final exams, I was given the opportunity to shadow an infusion nurse. Ellen became a teacher and a mentor. As I watched her care for patients in the infusion room, I grew to respect and admire not only her technical nursing skills but her gentle, caring spirit as well.

That was the beginning of our relationship. I continued to observe as Ellen led by example. Her gentle, calming spirit is an encouragement to all of the nurses in the outpatient infusion room. In my new role as a clinic nurse, Ellen and I often share care for patients. Many of my patients would request that Ellen be the treating nurse. We both became involved in their lives, and long after treatment ended, I would get a call from Ellen inquiring whether we had seen a specific patient and how he or she was doing. Too often, we have shared tears over patients for whom we no longer had an effective treatment.

Ellen cheered me on as I wrote and published the story of my daughter's survival of childhood cancer. When I was diagnosed with breast cancer, she and my other co-workers prayed and supported me as I continued to work while undergoing surgery and radiation therapy. The love and care I received sustained me.

Ellen quietly exhibits all the characteristics that make her an extraordinary nurse. She is proficient in her nursing skills, making her patients feel safe while in her care. She cares about all the things that are important to each individual, making them feel valued and loved. She celebrates small victories during the course of treatment. She remembers the little things that are important to the patient and family members. Though days can be harried and stressful, her gentle, quiet demeanor is a calming influence on both patients and staff. Even on the most difficult days, she maintains a positive attitude. While Ellen is one of the most soft-spoken persons I have ever known, her actions shout as she is on the front line of the battle with the patients she serves. She has a profound effect on her patients, their families, and her colleagues. She is an example of the kind of oncology nurse I aspire to be! ❧

TEACHING MOMENT:

She is proficient in her nursing skills, making her patients feel safe while in her care. She cares about all the things that are important to each individual, making them feel valued and loved.

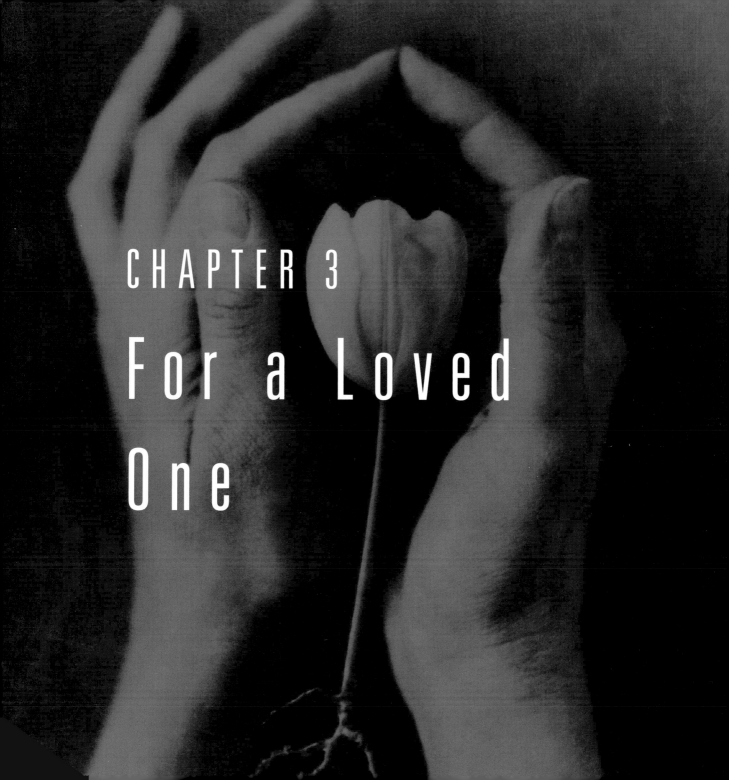

CHAPTER 3
For a Loved One

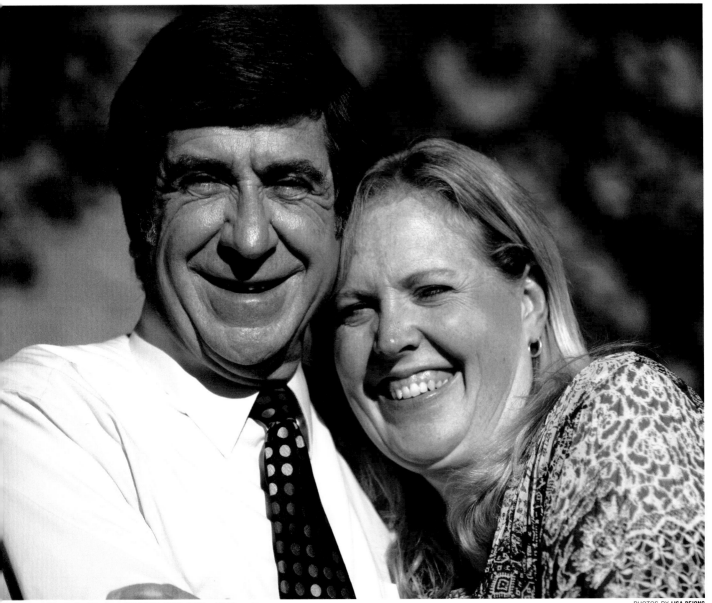

Machelle Moeller, RN, MSN, CNP, OCN, with Dave Day

Best of the Best

MACHELLE MOELLER, RN, MSN, CNP, OCN [CLEVELAND CLINIC IN CLEVELAND, OHIO]

WRITTEN BY DAVE DAY

LET ME FIRST state that *all* oncology nurses are angels. How blessed we are that they answer their calling to serve others when it's most needed.

MY WIFE'S JOURNEY with breast cancer began in June 2000. Although they had just met, Machelle Moeller was with her every step of the way—through surgery, initial radiation, and chemotherapy treatments. Weekly treatments continued, followed by more surgeries and rounds of radiation. Through the whole journey, Machelle continually went above and beyond the call of duty to ensure Suzanne's comfort and understanding of the procedures being done. They immediately bonded and became an inspiration to each other. As the spouse and caregiver, it melted my heart to see this. I can never repay Machelle for the professionalism, compassion, and love she gave Suzanne (and other patients at the Cleveland Clinic) throughout this journey. She was always there for Suzanne, always there for me, and always there for our sons.

In March 2009, my wife, Suzanne, passed away. Although it was almost nine years in the making, in one flash of a second, I lost my wife of 33 years, my soul-mate, my best friend, my inspiration, and the mother of our three boys. To her last breath, she continued to say that having breast cancer was actually a blessing. As she always put it, "Look at all the wonderful people that came into my life—who we otherwise may have never met." She truly meant this. Machelle was at the top of the list. How blessed we were to have such a wonderful guide along such a confusing and scary trail. On that same day in March, Machelle lost a dear friend. Our hearts are broken.

Cancer is a horrible and ugly disease. The patients who wake up every morning and put on "the armor" to battle this beast are the true heroes in this world. Those who help them (both physically and emotionally) on this journey are the angels we call oncology nurses. Machelle is the model of love, compassion, and dedication

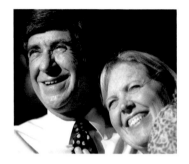

to both profession and patients. She will always mean the world to our family, and I, too, feel blessed that she came into our lives. May God continue to bless those individuals facing cancer head-on, those who tirelessly work to find a cure, and oncology doctors and nurses who dedicate their lives to care for others. The world is a good place—and Machelle is the best of the best. ❧

TEACHING MOMENT:

Through the whole journey, Machelle continually went above and beyond the call of duty to ensure Suzanne's comfort and understanding of the procedures being done.

Our Adopted Daughter

JANELL BONTRAGER, RN, BSN [GOSHEN CENTER FOR CANCER CARE IN GOSHEN, INDIANA]

WRITTEN BY TONY MCNAIR

For a
Loved One

SOMETIMES LIFE TURNS on a dime. Married for 44 years, Ann and I lived a careful, healthy lifestyle, planning to live to 120 and then turn out the lights. Melanoma changed our plans forever.

CANCER CHANGES your life. It takes you to a different place, and we were in our first days in that new place. We checked in at the Goshen Center for Cancer Care for treatment. Other than for childbirth, this was Ann's first hospitalization. An induced near-death experience is a tough introduction. In walked Janell Bontrager. She smiled and said, "I will be your nurse." Her simple statement expressed everything we needed to know. It was a perfect mix of total compassion and reassuring expertise. She promptly became our adopted daughter.

People have entered our lives in categories that don't have names. I call them adopted daughters and semi-cousins, but none shows the mixture of expertise, talent, friendship, and love that Janell brought to us in this ultimate time of need. She knew her nursing like an artist, but she also exuded care, concern, compassion, and joy. Of course, Janell didn't work 24 hours a day, but her presence was always felt in the room.

From beginning to end, Janell gave us totally devoted attention. I know she was giving the same service to her other patients, but it felt like we were the only patients in her world. Ann wanted to know about everyone's life, family, and interests. Janell told me later that the nurses scheduled 10 to 15 extra minutes with Ann because she always had questions and wanted to know more about their lives and families. But Janell was always there with answers, medical or personal.

Later, after we had to abandon that treatment, Ann was put on another chemotherapy. She had been well enough that we made a vacation trip to Yellowstone. Janell made a trip to Ireland. We ran into Janell and she wanted to see Ann's pictures from our trip. Ann told her we would be back on Friday. "That's my day off." One beat pause, and then she said, "I'll be here at 9:00; be sure you bring your pictures." Janell was there at 8:00 visiting with her other patients and friends. Once Ann was settled and they were talking, I left. I came back at noon; they were still talking. I took them to lunch and finally had to separate them so we could go home ... all on Janell's day off.

My wife passed away on May 9, 2008, after a 13-month battle. For all but the last four days, she had reason to hope and the spirit to fight. Cancer is such a senseless disease, but Ann (and I) looked forward to every visit to the Goshen Center in large part because of Janell's attitude, strength, and faith. Sadly, there was no silver bullet for us. We lost the battle, but in some ways, I have to say, we won the war. It was perhaps the best year Ann and I had together, and Janell was a big part of that. How can you find joy in cancer? By partnering with someone who unblinkingly looks cancer in the eye and does everything that is humanly possible for her patients.

She knew her nursing like an artist, but she also exuded care, concern, compassion, and joy.

I personally asked Janell and other Goshen staff to attend Ann's memorial service. It was both a tragic evening and a magical evening. Ann would have loved the party. When, toward the end of the service, I walked to the front to share my thoughts, the doors opened and in came Janell with two other nurses. They couldn't join us earlier because they had worked that afternoon, but their delayed entry let me bring them to the front and introduce them to everyone. It's an exceptional moment when you can put your arms around three angels at one time.

Without the Goshen Center for Cancer Care, we would have had six terrifying months together instead of 13 warm and memorable months. Without Janell Bontrager, it would have been an infinitely more difficult process. ❧

A Friend for Life

DANIEL VANDERGAST, RN, BSN [GREATER PHILADELPHIA HEMATOLOGY/ONCOLOGY IN PHILADELPHIA, PENNSYLVANIA]   WRITTEN BY BARBARA MICHALSKI

DAN IS A NURSE whom you can connect with immediately. My husband, Lee, was diagnosed in 2000 with non-Hodgkin lymphoma and was immediately scheduled for treatment for two types of large cell and small cell lymphoma. He was in the treatment room on Thursdays and Fridays, every 21 days. Somewhere in between those 21 days, there was always some sort of side effect from the chemo that meant he needed to go to the oncologist's office. Dan was a male nurse among an all-female staff, and when Lee and Dan first met, they immediately connected with one word—fishing.

For a
Loved One

DAN LOVED FISHING as much as Lee did, and they would talk about trips they made, what kind of fish they caught, what was biting, and what kind of bait to use. Lee always had fishing tips for people, and when Dan asked how to catch a certain kind of fish, Lee got his hooks and line, took them to the chemo unit, and showed Dan how to tie certain knots for catching fish.

It was definitely a place Lee did not want to be for six years, but Dan was the nurse who helped you get through those long chemo days and always gave you some suggestions on things for side effects from the chemo. If you were having any problems, he would interrupt the doctor (who might be seeing patients) if it was urgent enough. Dan would never let things you might think too small to mention go unattended.

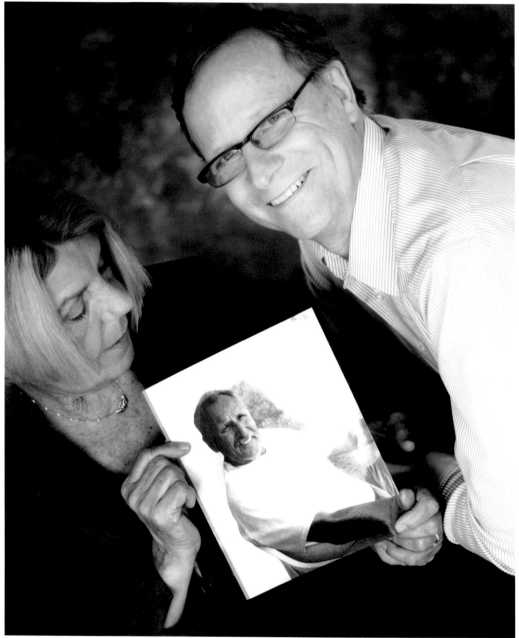

Daniel VanderGast, RN, BSN, with Barbara Michalski

He always had a hug for me and handshake for Lee, and his contagious smile and laugh always took your worried mind to another place. Once you meet him, you feel you have known him all your life. He was there at a phone call when Lee went into the hospital for the last time, and he attended Lee's funeral services with his wife. He truly had an impact on Lee, and his connection with his patients, doctors, and coworkers is excellent.

I believe God sends angels like Dan on a special mission to bring friendship and comfort to the sick and their families. He might not ever be aware of the enormous impact his heart puts out, but I know he will always be in my heart. ✤

TEACHING MOMENT:

Dan would never let things you might think too small to mention go unattended. He always had a hug for me and handshake for Lee, and his contagious smile and laugh always took your worried mind to another place.

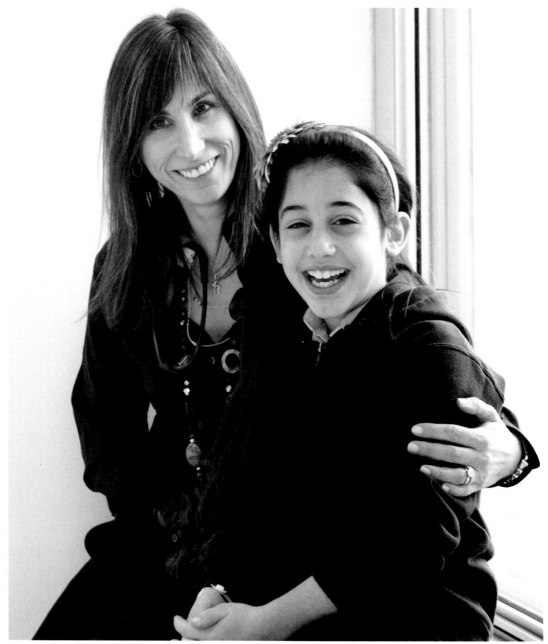

Jacquie Toia, RN, DNP, MS, with Rena Miller

Her Best Friend

JACQUIE TOIA, RN, DNP, MS [CHILDREN'S MEMORIAL HOSPITAL IN CHICAGO, ILLINIOS]

WRITTEN BY DANYA MILLER

WE WALKED OUT of the procedure suite—pale, heartbroken, downtrodden, and confused. Our six-year-old daughter, Rena, was just taken in for a bone marrow aspirate and spinal tap. We were unable to make any sense of what was going on. Rena, our second daughter, had just been diagnosed with leukemia. What type? What treatment? What risk level? What to expect? We had no idea. We had been assigned an oncologist in the ER the night before, and it was time to meet her.

WE SAT IN a small meeting room—two anxious, red-eyed parents, the doctor, and a resident. In comes Jacquie. "Hi guys! Sorry I'm late," Jacquie announced with a smile, catching her breath. She took a seat next to Dr. Morgan and folded her legs up under her like a pretzel, cowboy boots and all. Dr. Morgan turned to us with a half grin and said, "When Jacquie comes in she makes a statement." We gave a little chuckle, not knowing who Jacquie was or what impact she would have on this nightmare.

We soon found out that Jacquie is Dr. Morgan's nurse practitioner. According to Jacquie, they have been together so long that they are like an "old married couple." After Dr. Morgan explained to us that Rena had acute lymphoblastic leukemia and what its implications would be, she gave the floor to Jacquie. Exuding confidence, Jacquie described what typically happens to "her kids" throughout treatment. She spoke with clarity, in terms that we could understand. While she was very straightforward and did not hide any facts or statistics, the longer she spoke, the calmer we felt. Her casual demeanor and relaxed attitude instilled a feeling of trust—a feeling that has only grown stronger since then.

Throughout our first meeting, Jacquie assured us many times that she was always available, whether by pager, personal cell phone, or in person. We have taken advantage of all three. One night, Rena was in the emergency room, and Jacquie was scheduled to go on an international vacation early the next morning. We had called her to keep her apprised of the situation—not because she *needed* to know, but because *we* felt that we wanted to be in touch. Before hanging up she said, "Call me back when you're headed home; I'm curious about the outcome. It doesn't matter what time you call; I'll answer all night."

At one point, when Rena was an inpatient, Jacquie came into the room to give us results from a test. As soon as she came in, I said, "Oh, Jacquie, I am so glad to see you." She must have been able to read my face because she immediately took me into a side room and sat me down and said, "What's up?" That's all it took for the dam to break and the flood of tears to overflow. She sat with me for what seemed like an hour and calmly reviewed all the information she had already given us. The more she spoke, the calmer I felt. She never once said not to worry, that everything would be okay, and therefore, I knew I could believe her. She wasn't just trying to pacify me, and that was a tremendous comfort.

We've known Jacquie now for more than three years. We appreciate who she is and the impact she has had on all of us. She has bent over backward to make Rena as comfortable as possible, from pulling strings to get her into a procedure early, to asking her to teach her something that she has learned in school; from singing her favorite song during a spinal tap, to sneaking Rena an extra prize or two. As soon as Jacquie spots Rena at the clinic, she calls out, "Hey, Rena Bena! How ya' doin'?" Jacquie has made Rena feel like she's her favorite patient, but *all* of Jacquie's patients feel like that. She wouldn't have directed summer camp for children with cancer for more than two decades if she weren't loved by all.

But the best part about Jacquie is how much Rena loves her. Rena met Jacquie when she was at her worst—tired, irritable, hungry, in pain, and just plain miserable. For the first month, Rena wouldn't even speak to her. Jacquie has personally given Rena all of her spinal taps, has examined her in all kinds of embarrassing places, poked and prodded when unwanted, and prescribed all of the medicine that makes her so ill, yet Rena sums it up so eloquently: "I'm happy that I only have to go the clinic once a month now, but I'm sad about one thing. I won't get to see Jacquie so much. She is my best friend." ❧

A Bond of Love

JAIME SMITH, RN, BSN, OCN [PERRY COUNTY MEMORIAL HOSPITAL IN TELL CITY, INDIANA]

WRITTEN BY JAMES STAFFORD

"I LOVED HER." That is what Jaime Smith said to me at my wife Angie's funeral.

WE FIRST met nurse Jaime, head of the oncology nurses and the oncology team at Perry County Memorial Hospital, in April 2005, about four weeks after Angie's mastectomy. She was apologetic for the diagnosis as if it were her fault, but assured us that they would do everything they could to make Angie's treatments as comfortable as they could. At her sixth and final treatment, Jaime made sure there were banners and balloons celebrating the end of her treatment and the start of the rest of her life.

Less than a year later, we were back in her care after Angie's second diagnosis, this one worse than the first. As treatments progressed, Angie seemed to become more than just another patient to Jaime. She made sure that she was the one taking personal care of Angie. She always made sure we knew exactly what was going on, even when we couldn't understand the doctor or all the technical mumbo-jumbo. Even when we needed help with other doctors at other facilities, she went out of her way to spearhead the effort to get us what we needed. After Angie's surgery to remove the second tumor in as many years, it was back to routine checkups in the PCMH oncology department. Things were going well for more than a year, then in 2007, Jamie was the one to deliver Angie's final diagnosis. It was as if she had to tell her own sister or mother that they had cancer. She was as angry about the diagnosis as we were. Had we not done everything we could? She assured us that we did.

That news was delivered in October. Over the next year, Angie had many complications due to her breast cancer metastasizing to her brain. Jaime was instrumental in getting us appointments when there were no openings and tests or scans done when the machines were already full. She always made us feel like we were more important than anyone else and that we deserved preferential treatment.

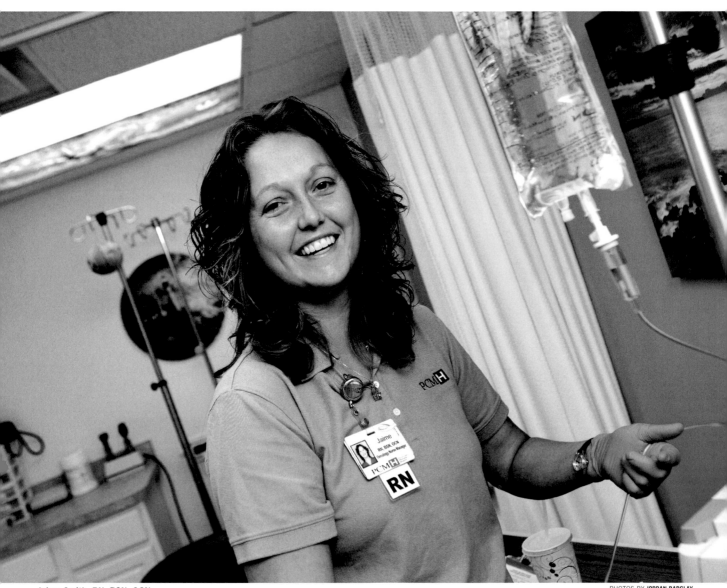

Jaime Smith, RN, BSN, OCN

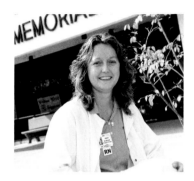

On November 22, 2008, three years and nine months after her first diagnosis, Angie passed away. It was a Saturday. At the funeral home on that next Monday, Jaime walked up to the casket and then to me. I expressed my sincerest thanks for everything she had done for Angie and for me. To this, she replied, "I loved her."

As the husband of a former patient, this meant more to me than any technical skill any medical care professional could ever display. ❧

TEACHING MOMENT:

She made sure that she was the one taking personal care of Angie. She always made sure we knew exactly what was going on, even when we couldn't understand the doctor or all the technical mumbo-jumbo.

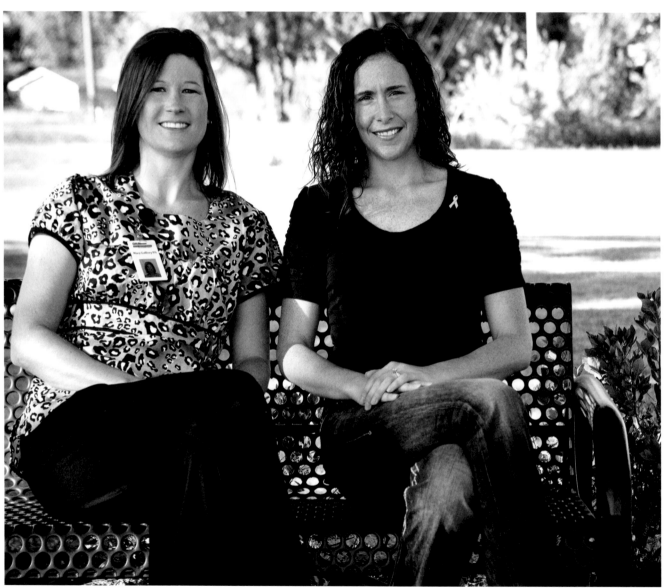

Mary Gaffney, RN [left] with Amy Heil Buechler

Saving a Life

MARY GAFFNEY, RN [ONCOLOGY HEMATOLOGY ASSOCIATES IN EVANSVILLE, INDIANA]

WRITTEN BY AMY HEIL BUECHLER

MY FATHER was diagnosed with bladder cancer in December 2008. He had surgery on January 23, 2009. It was at that time we were told it was small cell carcinoma of the bladder, which is a very rare type of bladder cancer, and that he would need chemotherapy.

For a
Loved One

WHEN HE CAME HOME from the hospital, he was still in a great deal of pain and eventually ended up back in the hospital with a tumor in his pelvis that had shut down his kidneys. At that point, stents were placed in to bypass his kidneys, and chemotherapy was started in the hospital. He was released from the hospital after three weeks, and he started chemotherapy the next day at Oncology Hematology Associates.

When my dad went to chemotherapy, it was a family affair. My mother, sister, and I went to show support, as we are an extremely close family. I will never forget meeting Mary. When she got the first bag of medication going, she told us that, if we needed anything, to let her know. I had no idea she really meant it. Throughout this time, she showed us the compassion and care one person could give. Not only did I see her give it to my father, but she also treated all of her other patients the same way. She would go out of her way to help us and always make sure our questions were answered.

This time was very hard for me in particular because I am extremely close to my dad. Mary told me she was there for me, and if she could ever do anything, she would be happy to. At that time, she gave me the phone number to her office to bypass the automated system and her cell phone number. There came a time when I had to take my dad to his chemotherapy appointment, but I couldn't stay. I wasn't worried at all because I knew Mary would take great care of my dad and that she would call me if I needed to get back there.

———

There came a time through the chemotherapy when my dad started having scans to check the progress of the chemotherapy. Each time my dad had a scan, we would have to wait a few days for the results. Waiting for the results caused me so much anxiety, I couldn't sleep at night, and I would get sick. Mary began calling to get the scan results only hours after the scan was completed. This became something she did for my family for every scan, even when my dad went into remission. She will never truly know the peace of mind her being there gave us.

Any time my dad was having any problems, I knew I could call Mary, and she would take care of it. One day, I had to call her because my father was having pain, and she called and had his routine scan moved up. It was a Friday afternoon, and she told the office the scan needed to be done "ASAP." It was rescheduled for Monday morning, but it was the week of spring break, so I knew we would not be able to get the results for a while. Mary called me and said she was going on a family vacation to Florida, but to call her when the scan was over, and she would still call and get the results. I could not believe she was still willing to take care of my family while she was on vacation with hers.

I called her when the scan was over, and she said she would let me know as soon as the results were in. A few hours later, she had another nurse call us and let us know that, indeed, there was a mass in my dad's abdomen. This nurse read the radiology report to me and let me know our oncologist was on vacation and would not be back until Friday morning. The tumor had grown considerably in three months. It was already 9 cm by 6.5 cm. All we thought was "Can it wait that long?" Mary contacted one of the other oncologists in the practice and asked him for a personal favor—to see us the very next day. He agreed to do it. From that point, the ball was rolling, and my dad started radiation that week.

If Mary had not been willing to take time out of her vacation, who knows how long it would have taken us to get the results of the scan, see our oncologist, see the radiation oncologist, have the radiation simulation, and begin radiation. I truly believe Mary saved my father's life.

Mary showed us what one person who cares can do. I now think of Mary as a part of my family and wish that one day I can repay her for her kindness and compassion. She has a very special place in my heart and is the most wonderful, caring person I have ever met! ❧

Beacon of Hope

ROBIN BRENDEL, BSN, OCN [MEMORIAL SLOAN-KETTERING CANCER CENTER IN ROCKVILLE CENTRE, NEW YORK]   WRITTEN BY ROBIN DONOVAN

MY HUSBAND Bill's journey began in October 2009 when he was diagnosed with stage 4, squamous cell carcinoma of the neck. We chose Memorial Sloan-Kettering Cancer Center (MSKCC). The fact they have a Long Island campus was instrumental in our final decision because Bill could receive treatment close to where we live. We felt we made the right decision, but we did not know what was in store for us.

ROBIN BRENDEL works as an oncology nurse in the outpatient facility at MSKCC of Rockville Centre (located in western Nassau County) that includes chemotherapy and radiation therapy. Robin proved to be our "beacon of hope" in our odyssey. After the second week of six weeks' worth of scheduled visits of chemotherapy and radiation, Bill was cooking dinner and eating with the family. After the third week, Bill's frame of mind changed. He did not feel good. He ended up in the hospital. He was still able to make his appointments because MSKCC is located on the grounds of Mercy Hospital. It was a short wheelchair ride away.

During this week—when Bill was in the hospital—I met Robin in the outpatient facility. Robin was there to relate her experience, strength, and hope with us. Her husband, a survivor, had been diagnosed with the same stage 4, squamous cell carcinoma as Bill's only five years earlier. On the day she shared this with us, our lives began to change. "How was this possible?" I asked myself. The fact we were being cared for by an oncology nurse who had firsthand experience seemed more than coincidental. The first couple of times she mentioned how her husband was able to get through his regimen, I began to listen carefully, trust what she

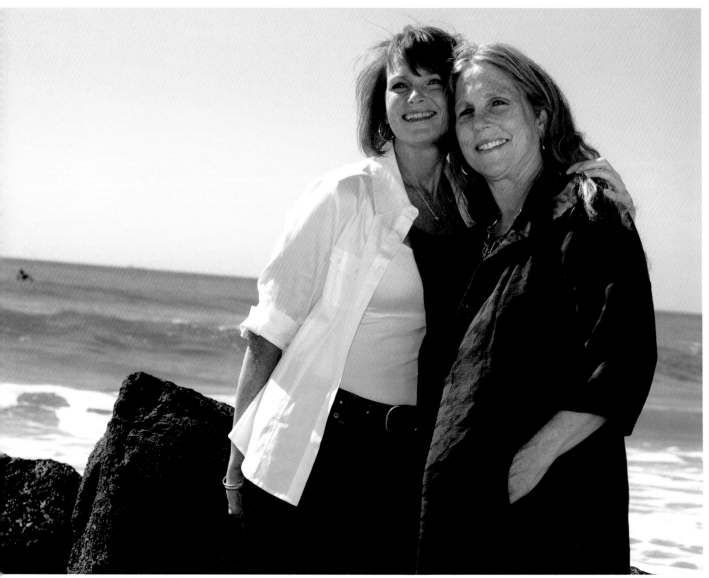

Robin Brendel, BSN, OCN [left] with Robin Donovan

had to say, and write down notes vigorously. I could tell she thought the world of her husband by the way she talked about him. She did not need to reveal too much, but just enough to make Bill and me comfortable with what was happening to us. She always referred to her husband while attending to my husband. Every time we heard her husband's name, we felt uplifted. It was as if she were a beacon, shining on us, leading our way out of the darkness. We looked forward to seeing her, receiving her gentle care, and listening to her words of wisdom.

Robin's wonderful healing tips not only included emotional care but also her uncanny ability to pinpoint what was needed at any particular moment. With myriad medications that seemed to change frequently, she was able to ascertain what to do. When I told her that Bill was not taking one of his medications, she told us that her husband felt the same way at times. That gave us hope and encouragement to keep going. She explained to us that, because of all the radiation that had been administered to Bill's throat, he needed to take his pain medication because he was not aware of how much pain he was in, due to the fact he could not swallow. This was also important because, ultimately, he would need to practice swallowing exercises routinely.

Having a feeding tube was not an easy thing to get used to either. Bill was curious to know when Robin's husband was able to start eating solid foods again. Robin explained that, due to the radiation, her husband wasn't able to eat steak until six months after his treatment ended. Bill was disappointed, but he also had something to look forward to.

One day Robin said to my husband, "You are beginning to look like the person who first came in to us. I can see the sparkle in your eyes." It was so wonderful to see Bill smile when he heard this. Bill is now on the road to recovery. Each day he gets a little stronger. I know he is eager to get back to doing the things he has done before, and we realize it is going to take time.

Robin's insight helped us gain a perspective on the short- and long-term goals we could hope to achieve in the future. Her experience gave us a sense of security and serenity. What we learned from Robin, we knew we could implement at home on a daily basis and even help someone else in a similar situation as ours. Robin inspired us to remain confident. The fact that her husband was a survivor was paramount. He became our "beacon of hope" as much as Robin. We knew Robin was as special to him as she was to us. ✖

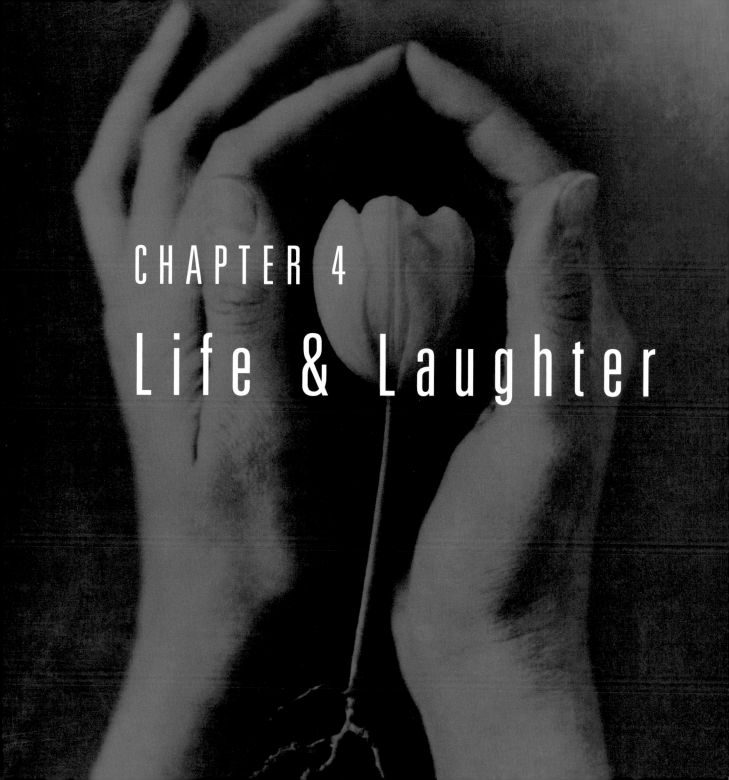

CHAPTER 4
Life & Laughter

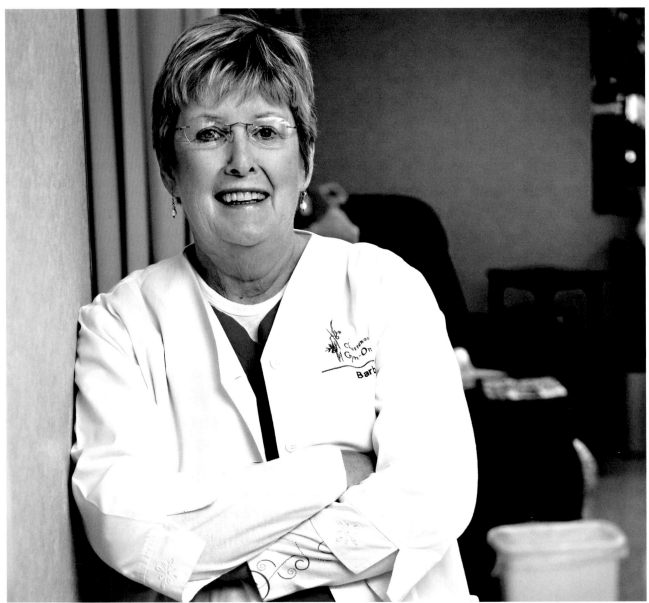

Barbara Perchalski, RN

Ready to Rumble

BARBARA PERCHALSKI, RN [CHATTANOOGA GYN-ONCOLOGY IN CHATTANOOGA, TENNESSEE]
WRITTEN BY MAUREEN WAGNER

BARBARA MAKES YOU FEEL at ease from the moment you walk into the chemo room. She relishes your ability to cope with chemo treatments and supports you every step of the way. I walked into my first chemo appointment with boxing gloves on to let everyone know I was "ready to rumble!" Barbara made sure all the other patients knew about it to inspire them to fight as hard as they can.

BARBARA NOTICED I was in pain during a treatment and made sure to call the doctor over to investigate. I had such pain in my back because there is a tumor on one of my nerves, and the pills they gave me just were not working. Thanks to Barbara, I now have a pain patch and am pain-free for the first time in weeks!

Barbara calls to remind me of appointments, to remember to give myself a shot, or just to say "hello" and see how I am getting along. I really feel like she is by my side every step of the way. She even indulges me when I bring in a martini glass to treatment and ask that my juice be served in the martini glass to make the treatment go a little easier.

Her desire is to see all of us well again. She knows each of us by name and makes sure we get to know each other, so we can help each other through the journey. Barbara makes treatment as enjoyable as it can be. She makes sure we take time to laugh and enjoy what we are all thankful for—we are surviving and will hopefully, one day, be cancer-free. ✤

Lifting Us Up

JAN HILDEBRANDT, RN [SURREY MEMORIAL HOSPITAL IN SURREY, BRITISH COLUMBIA, CANADA]

WRITTEN BY DANI MILLER

AT AGE 29, I was sitting alone in a hospital basement waiting for a MUGA scan in anticipation of a double mastectomy. Someone had just told me I had a heart murmur, and, oh yeah, they were going to cut off my boobs and do chemo, too.

I WAS TRYING really, really hard not to panic as I sat there waiting for the unknown, trying to act like I'd been doing this forever. It wasn't working very well. Five more minutes on my own, and I would have been a puddle on the floor. Thankfully, before I got to that point, my luck changed rather abruptly when Jan walked in.

Jan was in a nurse uniform, but she sat down to wait. I noticed her hair was really short (buzz), and she was waiting for a MUGA too. I took a stab and asked her, "Are you a cancer patient?" And my whole terribly scary experience was changed—for the better. Jan was a breast cancer survivor and had gone through everything I was about to. She also worked in the hospital I was at and was getting her MUGA on her lunch hour. Jan became my "guardian angel" as I started down the hardest path I have had to walk so far in this life.

Jan started right up front and assured me, with no end of spunk, this was not a death sentence. She comforted me and went to check her schedule for me. She is a surgical nurse who works with the team of doctors who specialize in breast cancer at my local cancer center. Jan came back happy to tell me I had great doctors lined up and she was my nurse for surgery that next day.

I went to sleep with Jan holding my hand and woke up laughing. She'd covered me in stickers. It's quite a thing to come out of anesthesia in post-op to find your boobs may be missing, but somebody has taken the time to put funny stickers all over you. I found stickers on my wrist band, my dressings, you name it. I laughed out loud despite it all.

Jan stuck with me. She taught me about chemo, taught me about doctors, tests, radiation, and held my hand for another surgery. She checked on me my first day of chemo, answered the phone whenever I called, e-mailed me, and came to my housewarming to celebrate life with me when I was done with radiation. Jan became my friend.

We are still in touch, two years later. I think the most amazing thing about Jan is that I know it's not just me. She chooses to work with breast cancer patients as much as she can. She works behind the scenes to help the hospital improve the experience whenever she can. She takes on each one of us she meets individually, holds us close, and lifts us up. That is an extraordinary healer! ❧

TEACHING MOMENT:

She checked on me my first day of chemo, answered the phone whenever I called, e-mailed me, and came to my housewarming to celebrate life with me when I was done with radiation. Jan became my friend.

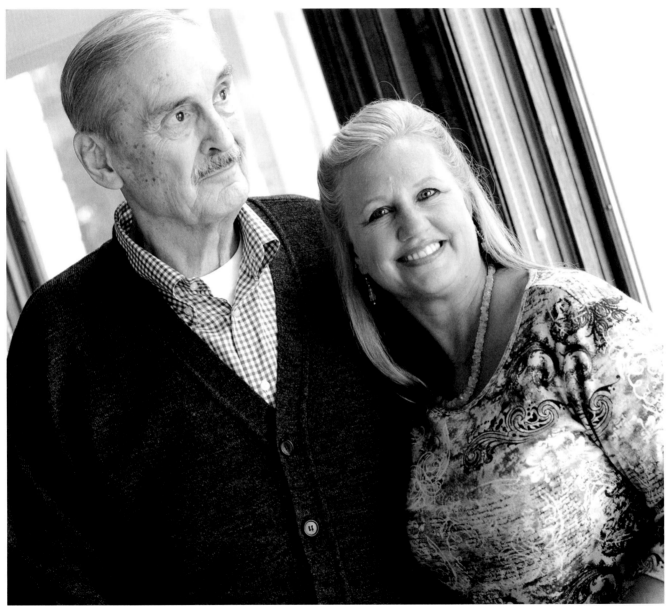

Janelle Kerns, RN, OCN, with Rainsford Brown

Sitting on the Fence

JANELLE KERNS, RN, OCN [IOWA CANCER SPECIALISTS IN BETTENDORF, IOWA]

WRITTEN BY RAINSFORD BROWN

THROUGHOUT LIFE, everyone experiences times of fence-sitting—not knowing which way to go. But for the cancer survivor, it often becomes a way of life. From that first diagnostic pronouncement of "you have cancer," the fence becomes an all too familiar stopping place. The unknown, the indecision, and the array of options make the fence a very uncomfortable and fearful place to reside. Waiting in the unknown for biopsy results, treatment regimens, prognosis reports, treatment progression, side effects, and test results adds to the misery. One's mind runs rampant during these times and can usually imagine the worst.

ENTER THE ONCOLOGY/INFUSION NURSE. I'm sure there are hundreds of wonderful Florence Nightingale–type nurses around the country fulfilling their calling, but I would highlight and honor Janelle Kerns. Janelle, for nearly five years in my continuing cancer battle, has not only taken care of all the medical issues with great professional efficiency but also has always helped provide me a way to climb down from that fence. Helpful information, informed choices, a listening ear, an encouraging hug, and just being there are the tools she supplies to assist in climbing off the fence. She also has a heart for the caregiver, knowing the strain and fatigue associated with the one standing by.

I've watched Janelle as she interacts with many other patients as well. She is knowledgeable, outgoing, on top of every detail of treatment and scheduling, compassionate, and truly caring. She is always willing to give or get an answer in the office or on the phone. She's never too busy and always returns calls when she says she will. She is truly an asset to the office of my wonderful, gifted, and brilliant oncologist who, together with Janelle, has kept me alive with treatment and hope.

I know many of her patients share in these feelings of gratitude for her personalized nursing; but for me, I applaud and appreciate Janelle for all of the attributes above, and most of all, for her human understanding of the pain of sitting on a fence. On top of that, she's cute—as an old codger, it's okay for me to say that, my wife says. ❧

TEACHING MOMENT:

She is always willing to give or get an answer in the office or on the phone. She's never too busy and always returns calls when she says she will. She is truly an asset to the office of my wonderful, gifted, and brilliant oncologist who, together with Janelle, has kept me alive with treatment and hope.

In the Trenches

SANDRA CANTY, RN, MS, OCN [ELMHURST MEMORIAL HEALTHCARE INFUSION CENTER IN ELMHURST, ILLINOIS]   WRITTEN BY KRISTINE KEDZIOR

THE WHOLE TEAM of oncology nurses at Elmhurst Memorial Healthcare Infusion Center is extraordinary. I admired the teamwork that was coordinated in my heath care. I appreciate all of the nurses who cared for me, and they each hold a special place in my heart.

IF I HAVE TO CHOOSE a primary care nurse, I would choose Sandra Canty because my chemotherapy started and ended with Sandy caring for me. That does not mean the other nurses were any less extraordinary. They were all exceptional, and they need to be honored as well.

I have to confess: I was terrified of chemo. I had to have a port for the protocol they followed for my chemotherapy. The oncology doctor reassured me this was minor, and in a few days following the surgery, I would be able to undergo chemo. All true. I thought it would be a walk in the park compared to having minor abdominal surgery requiring an incision that extended a few inches above my waist down to the pubic area. Wrong! Regardless of the size, it hurts when they cut your body. Because of the protocol, I had to have blood drawn 24 hours before chemo—that's when I first met Sandy. She was sensitive to the fact that the port was still sore. She thought it would be better to draw the blood from my vein. We chatted, and I began to feel better about the whole chemo business. Sandy gave me a hug and told me that she and I would see this thing through together. I had been fervently praying, "Please Lord no chemo, no chemo." Even though that didn't happen, I was sent these wonderful angels of mercy into my life.

Sandy always remembered I liked to sit in one corner in the main part of the room. When I would arrive early in the morning on Thursday, as soon as she saw me, she'd tell me to go ahead—my place was ready.

Sandy, as well as the other nurses, was so careful with the drugs. They checked, and then double-checked with another nurse. I really appreciated that. After all, I knew these weren't some fancy, feel good drugs they were pumping into my veins. They were poison, killer drugs. I was concerned about their contact with needles, the blood, and the poison, but they were always so careful. They were always quick to respond to the beeping of the machine, to switch to the next drug, so that I could get out of there as quickly as humanly possible. If my nurse for that day was busy, one of the other nurses would help out. Great teamwork! They kept a close eye on me too. I remember one time I looked up from what I was doing (I always brought some sewing or another project I was working on, my current book I was reading, a coffee drink, and a snack), and I saw Sandy looking at me. When our eyes met, she asked me if I needed something. I said, "No, you were the one looking at me." We laughed over that.

TEACHING MOMENT:

When our eyes met, she asked me if I needed something. I said "No, you were the one looking at me." We laughed over that.

Sandy patiently taught me about the pump I had to wear for 48 hours. Boy, did we have a time with that belt. I had been petite before the cancer, so during the chemo there was not much left of me. That belt was huge, but of course Sandy showed me how to make it work. Sandy knew I wanted to be informed, so she always gave me a copy of the results of my blood and urine tests. She'd answer my questions and give advice I was able to relate to. Her philosophy was: if it didn't hurt you and it helped, it was okay. She said if it didn't bother you to eat Mexican food, go ahead—just eat. When my potassium and salt were low, we decided chips and soda would work. Her approach to dietary problems just made more sense to me. I am so thankful for everything the nurses did for me. When the nurses would tell me something, I believed them. They reached me on a level I could relate to. The doctors were wonderful, but they were like the generals coordinating the war plans. The nurses were the soldiers in the trenches with me, waging the war against cancer.

What a relief when I finished chemo. I never thought I'd finish. I received a certificate and everything. I hugged Sandy and reminded her she had said we would make it through together, and we had. ❧

The Good "C"

CAROL LIEBAN, RN, BSN, OCN [QUEEN'S MEDICAL CENTER IN HONOLULU, HAWAII]

WRITTEN BY JERI GERTZ

I HAD BEEN contemplating the letter "C" as it applied to my husband's life—cancer, carcinoma, chemotherapy—when she walked in.

GROWING UP, I heard adults whisper about cancer as "the big, bad C" like a wolf whose name was too fearsome to utter aloud. I babysat for kids glued to *Sesame Street*, a television program sometimes "brought to you by the letter C," but they were always carefree words, like chocolate or carnival—never cancer.

It was February 11, 2003, Jim's first day in Queen's Medical Center in Honolulu. She walked into his room and said she would be Jim's primary nurse. She introduced herself as Carol.

"Aloha, Carol, are you a *good* C or a *bad* C?" I asked, trying to find a warm way to work with the cold reality of my husband's situation. With a cheerful confidence we came to know and love, Carol replied, "I'm a *good* C, and I guess you know you're not in Kansas anymore!"

She was right. We were strangers in the strange land called cancer. Only two weeks earlier, Jim had been diagnosed with inoperable, stage 4, pharyngeal carcinoma. It felt like everything was being brought to us by the letter C, and all of it felt like a calamity.

Enter Carol, with her caring, capable ways. She was of compact stature and immense skills, with clear, cerulean eyes. Carol had been an oncology nurse for more than 30 years, attended to thousands of patients, and yet she continually listened and compassionately responded to our concerns, as if it was the first time she was ever hearing them. She was a wise and gentle interpreter in that foreign land.

Jim was a guest of the oncology ward from February through August, so he was never in the hospital during the Christmas season, but was treated to plenty of what I came to call "Carol-ing." Carol spread her good cheer and excellent care to every patient and caregiver on the ward. She was completely dedicated and

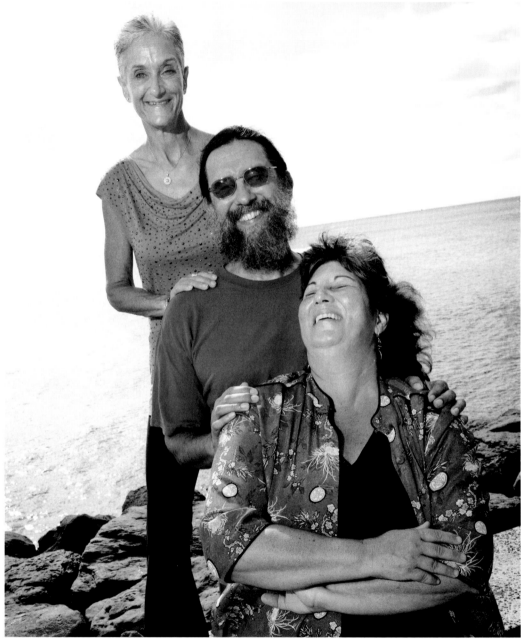

Carol Lieban, RN, BSN, OCN [top] with Jim and Jeri Gertz

often consulted by doctors for her opinions. Carol chose not to ascend to higher levels of nursing administration because of her passion for direct patient care.

Here are just a few shining examples of Carol's bright constellation.

In the middle of treatment, an MRI revealed the tumors at the base of Jim's brain continued to grow, despite concurrent radiation and chemotherapy. Carol helped us cope with the undiluted fear that was growing even faster than the cancer. She had a way of speaking and listening with equal intensity, and of offering informed hope. Carol helped make the best of things in the worst of times.

When I was frightened by Jim's medication-induced hallucinations, Carol brought comfort. She had seen such scenarios before and said Jim would have no memory of the incidents. He didn't. More important, Carol helped me realize that it did no good for me to retain disturbing images that for Jim were nonexistent. She helped us shed what we didn't need and offered wisdom and skills that we desperately needed in the struggles we faced. Carol was a nurse, a counselor, and a patient advocate to the bone.

One image we all happily retain is of Jim's final chemo bag. Carol decorated it with cheerful flower stickers. She called her creative handiwork "the aloha bag," referencing the multiple word meaning of *hello, goodbye, and love*. Her dedicated gaze glowed as she connected it to Jim's I.V. line.

I am grateful beyond words that Carol was assigned to us that first day. And I do mean *us*. Throughout the eight grueling months of Jim's treatment, we were both lucky recipients of Carol's high-caliber care. She was Jim's medical go-to champion and my communing co-pilot, helping me chart a careful course across cancerous skies. If oncology nursing was an Olympic event—and I certainly think it qualifies—Carol would take the gold in every category.

Jim is now a glorious six years into remission, and our contact with Carol has moved outside the hospital—to beaches, hikes on our island's lava flows, and to Scrabble games. Although it was planted in a medical crisis, we now enjoy a healthy garden of continually blooming friendship with this extraordinary healer. Carol will always be the *good* C—a comrade who was there in the clutch. We're grateful that she continues to share her incomparable character. ❧

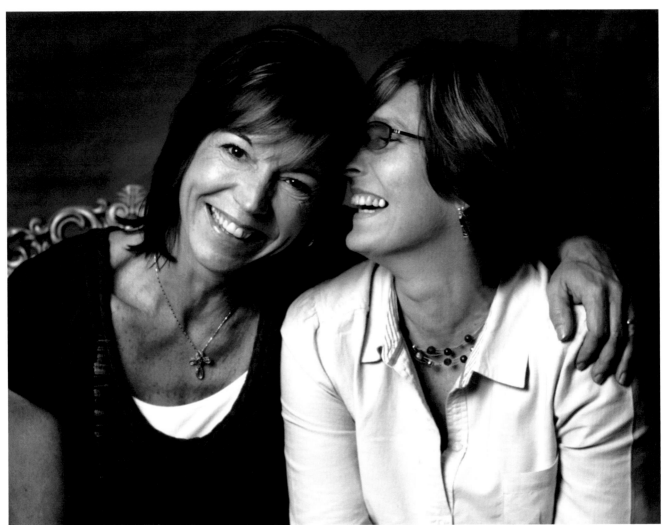

Carolanne Wismer, RN, OCN [left] with Dianne Killian

Supernatural

CAROLANNE WISMER, RN, OCN [FOX CHASE CANCER CENTER IN PHILADELPHIA, PENNSYLVANIA]

WRITTEN BY DIANNE KILLIAN

CAROLANNE WISMER is not just a nurse, she's a *great* nurse! There were many nurses we met, but we know she's the one! Her years of endless dedication to her patients far surpass what is expected from any nurse. She has super powers—we're sure of it. There are so many wonderful adjectives we could use to describe her, but unselfish and tireless in her duty to the name of nursing are what most stand out.

BILL, I, AND OUR FAMILIES do not know where we would have been without her sacrifice of giving the extra effort and time, or the tender way she guided us when we were so overwhelmed with the diagnosis of cancer. Her genuine compassion for sharing every bit of herself, assisting us in coping with the programs ahead, such as the lab, the infusion, X-rays, doctors, medications, and diet—this was all new to us, but not to her. She knows how to help, and she does almost immediately on first contact. She makes it her priority to help patients understand so they can better handle their role in working to get to a better place. And she does it with such ease, care, and with a great sense of humor.

I have been witness to Carolanne showing this gift to all her patients. She has a way of making you feel that you are her one and only patient. This means so much to a patient and his or her family. Carolanne has gone above and beyond the call of duty as a nurse and has become part of the families she has helped who are living with cancer. We have looked to her for advice, to assist, to explain, and to be totally honest. And when she does tell you, she is not harsh.

Carolanne has never had a problem sharing the pain we feel. There are so many examples. The moments holding hair back when patients have to throw up—if they have hair—getting answers to questions no matter how trivial they might seem, making a meal, holding a hand, hugs, lots of hugs, fighting to get test results a little faster, or getting a patient in a little earlier for infusion. She will tell you something funny to bring your spirits up, listening to your fears, your dreams, your hopes. And she helps family members of cancer patients understand what to expect, explaining with care what the patient is going through. She takes time from her personal life and family to call just to see how your day is going or how you are feeling after chemo. She says, if there's anything she can do for you, to just call her no matter what time it is. Wow! She is really wow!

There are so many great nurses that we have met, know and have known at Fox Chase in our six years there, but we have never met anybody quite like

TEACHING MOMENT:

I have been witness to Carolanne showing this gift to all her patients. She has a way of making you feel that you are her one and only patient. This means so much to a patient and his or her family.

Carolanne in any hospital. When we didn't know which way to turn or which decision to make that would take a burden from our overwhelmed and confused lives dealing with cancer, she was there and still is.

She made it bearable. She made the impossible, possible and the hard times seem easier. She is the one—one in a million. ✤

Easing the Burden

PATTIE CONROY-VATALARO RN, BSN, OCN [ON CARE HAWAII IN HONOLULU, HAWAII]

WRITTEN BY BEVERLY GANTT

I HAVE FACED cancer four times in the past 28 years. Three of these times in the past 10 years, I've managed with courage and strength because of Pattie Conroy-Vatalaro.

I FIRST MET Pattie in 2000, when I went to my first chemotherapy session at Kuakini Hospital in Honolulu, Hawaii. I was very scared and apprehensive about what was going to happen. I was set for gloom and doom but was met instead by a smiling oncology nurse who walked me through my first chemo session. Her patience and expertise set my mind at ease. I came to realize that my weekly trips for chemo would not be as bad as I had envisioned.

In 2007 and 2009, my colorectal cancer metastasized, and I met up with Pattie again; this time she was working directly in my oncologist's office. She was located in a small private room, which had six infusion recliners and a small nurse's station.

Most of the time, all the chairs are filled with patients receiving infusions, receiving various booster shots, or getting their ports flushed. One might think that this is a truly overburdening job—one nurse, six patients, doctors in and out with orders and questions—but this is where Pattie shines.

Picture a short, blonde nurse—like a Disneyland employee or Alice in Wonderland at age 16—in bright colored scrubs, wearing a different colored Croc on each foot. I look forward to seeing her choice of colored Crocs or the latest doodads she has pinned on them, collections she picks up herself or receives from patients.

Don't be fooled by this picture. Pattie is super-competent in her role as an oncology nurse. She deals with

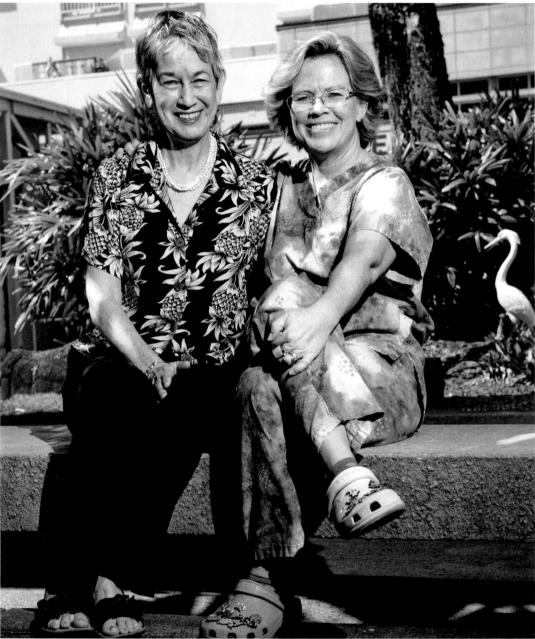

Pattie Conroy-Vatalaro, RN, BSN, OCN [right] with Beverly Gantt

each patient efficiently, quickly, with the utmost care and concern, and with expert knowledge and experience. This is "nurse" Pattie.

But I want to tell you about "friend" Pattie. Every patient is special to her. She remembers the type of chemo regimen you are on, the details of dosages, but most important, she remembers you. She knows what frightens you and what makes you smile, and this is what makes the chemo experience bearable.

Pattie inserts an I.V. in you while talking about how good the food looks on the flat screen in the room to distract you from your fear of needles. When your chemo gives you the runs, she is quick to give you more medicine to help you get through. She saves the recliner nearest the bathroom if you are inclined to frequent usage during chemo.

She treats you like a family friend. She tells you about her family and her week, and she remembers things you told her about you and your family. She does this all the while attending to your medical needs. She quickly answers the questions that you forget or are afraid to ask your doctor.

I have made about 120 visits to chemo over the years. Pattie always makes me feel at ease. Pattie's presence makes the process an easier burden to bear. Knowing her positive and friendly attitude will be there to help makes the trip more tolerable.

Pattie means the world to me in this journey with cancer, and I thank her for all she has done and continues to do for me and many others. ❧

TEACHING MOMENT:

Pattie's presence makes the process an easier burden to bear. Knowing her positive and friendly attitude will be there to help makes the trip more tolerable.

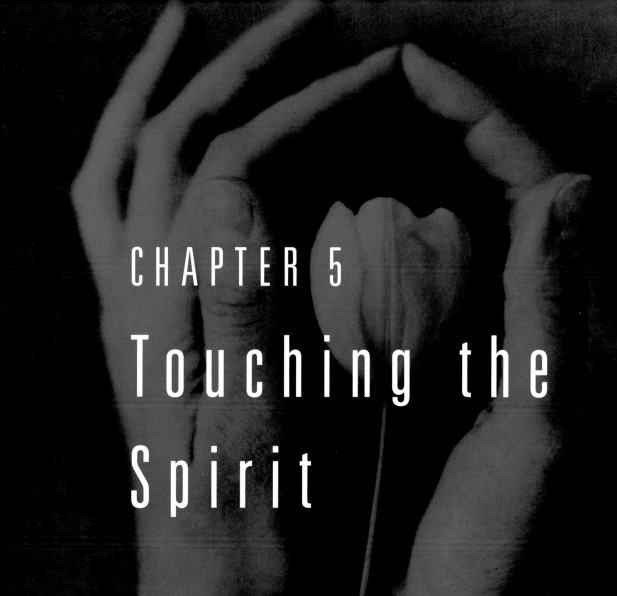

CHAPTER 5
Touching the
Spirit

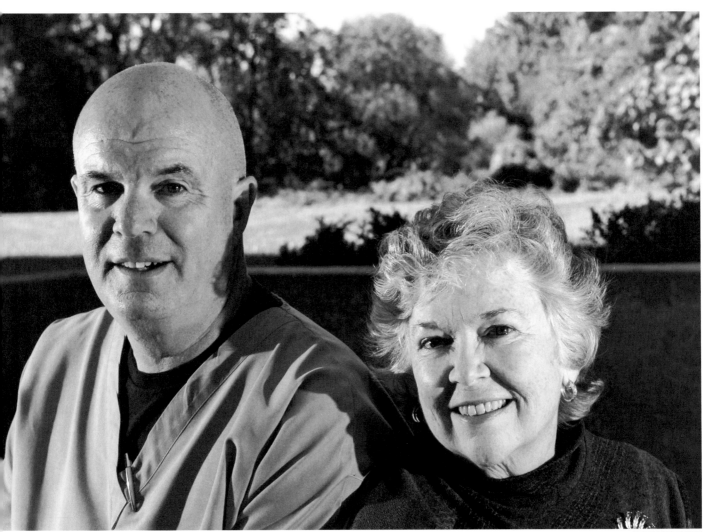

Ron Chubin, RN, OCN, with Charmaine L. Ciardi

Inspiring Strength

RON CHUBIN, RN, OCN [SHADY GROVE ONCOLOGY IN ROCKVILLE, MARYLAND]

WRITTEN BY CHARMAINE L. CIARDI

HAVING JUST completed my weekly treatments and feeling a little worn around the edges, I stopped downstairs at the pharmacy to get a new anti-nausea medication. As I picked it up, the pharmacist told me to wait, that my oncology nurse had called and was coming down. Two minutes later, with cup of water in one hand (to speed the ingestion of the new drug) and a prescription for another med that I needed in the other hand, Ron showed up to be sure that I got all of the help he could arrange. Extraordinary caring—typical of my long-term experiences with my nurse.

HE IS A BIG GUY with a shaved head and looks more like a drill sergeant or a lumberjack than a nurse. Like many big men, he moves with assurance, speaks with authority, and has a large presence. He has guided me through the vagaries of chemotherapy and living through life despite my metastatic disease. He does all of those professional things that are required of him—double-checks and then checks again to be sure I am getting the correct potion. He washes and washes and washes his hands. He keeps the schedule of my appointments and blood tests and scans, making sure that I am current. He calls to see if I am okay and that I can make my next treatment. He speaks to the doctors for me when needed and gets prescriptions for me when the pain is too much. He accesses and flushes my port. He monitors my weight, blood pressure, and temperature. He is my lifeline in this strange new world, as are all of his fellow oncology nurses. What is so special about him is the singular manner with which he protects and serves his patients.

Cancer not only assaults the body. It also attacks the soul. In an insidious way, it makes the patient feel vulnerable. In my case, my lifelong confidence has been leached away—my usual optimism seriously threatened. Cancer made me feel inadequate and diminished, fearful of what lies ahead.

Ron has made my weekly visits to him occasions wherein my spirit as well as my body has been treated. He relates to everyone with respect—his patients, their families, messengers, custodial staff, everybody. He remembers names, hobbies, trips, children, and spouses. He shares enough of himself that he is a vital presence to his patients, a force for healing. Along the way he banters, laughs, tells stories, learns more, and shares movie and restaurant reviews. He expects his patients to rise to meet him on the larger plane of shared humanity. And, despite the awful disease that brings us together, we do so. Ron has spent the better part of the last quarter of a century helping the sickest of the sick. He has told me all he ever wanted to do was help people, and that is his perfect job. I believe him. He works as if each patient is very personal to him. He really cares for us. And sitting there, watching the drip as he livens up the infusion center, we can feel his touch. He puts himself into overdrive on behalf of his patients, and we treasure him for it.

TEACHING MOMENT:

He expects his patients to rise to meet him on the larger plane of shared humanity.

I have never met a crabby oncology nurse. In the several-years-too-many that I have needed weekly treatments and on all the doctor's visits in between, I have yet to meet a nasty oncology nurse. They are a special breed, having chosen to work with really sick patients, many of whom can't win the fight before them. Day after day, these nurses show up smiling, caring, knowing, and helping. They share the tricks to ease the effects of toxic treatments, to help the belly, to soothe the mind. They encourage and support and mend. Their touch brings strength at a time when strength is on the wane. They are indeed a special bunch. They shine among humankind.

Ron is an extraordinary example of this incredible group. I attribute my own survival to date in no small measure to his strong, kind, competent, and gentle care. Ron Chubin is an extraordinary healer. ❧

Side by Side

DONNA BUSH, RN, OCN [NORTHWEST GEORGIA ONCOLOGY CENTER IN MARIETTA, GEORGIA]

WRITTEN BY HELEN TIPTON

I HAVE WATCHED Donna work with and support many patients in the past year, and I stand in awe of her ability to make everyone feel that their cancer journey is not a singular event. She is amazing to watch as she scurries around solving problems, soothing frayed nerves, and reassuring everyone she comes in contact with. From Northwest Georgia Oncology's standpoint, she must surely be the ultimate example of what they would hope each professional exemplifies. She demonstrates the highest imaginable energy level, the most positive and uplifting attitude, and yet is extremely professional while she continuously goes above and beyond all patient expectation.

THE MOST AMAZING thing about Donna, however, is how she makes me feel. Cancer is, of course, a universal problem and concern, but being diagnosed with it creates a very personal impact on the individual. From day one of my chemotherapy, I have considered Donna to be my nurse. Since she is a survivor herself, she can empathize with the constant torment and feelings of helplessness and anxiety that come with being diagnosed and treated for cancer.

Having been there herself, Donna can relate to the omnipresent concerns that go with the unknowns associated with the cancer diagnosis. Yes, it's treatable, but will my treatment work? How will my body react?

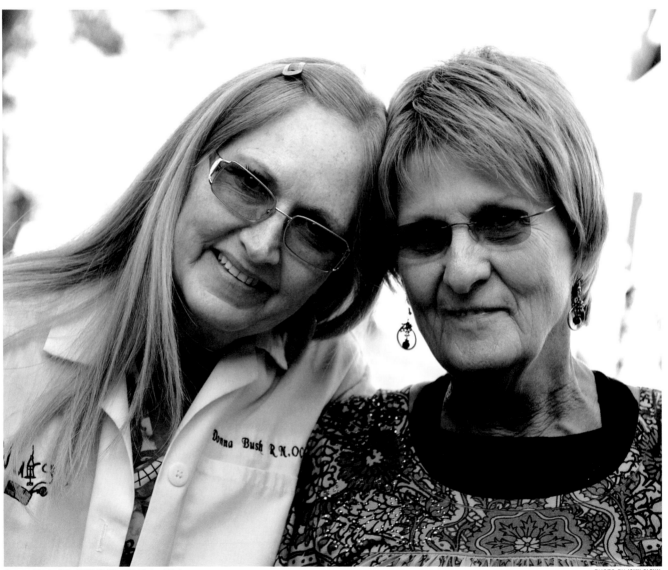

Donna Bush, RN, OCN [left] with Helen Tipton

Will I survive and, if so, how long? What about … and on and on. This is where Donna excels. She is constantly friendly, helpful, reassuring, and understanding. Because of my being on a research program, which caused me to have an exaggerated sense of euphoria, I required extra care and attention from Donna. She has always been extremely patient and taken the time to ensure my safety and comfort—whether going and coming to and from the restroom or getting down to the lobby for a ride home. Even though I tried to tell her I was all right, she stuck by my side without fail. Of course, no treatment day goes by without at least a hug or two. Even when I am not scheduled for treatment, if I come across her in the hall, elevator, or anywhere, Donna makes it a point to come over and ask how I am doing and always gives me that all-important healing hug. I swear, I felt like just having Donna as my nurse did me almost as much good as the chemotherapy. She is fun to be around and has a wonderful sense of humor to go along with her other qualities.

In summary, Donna has made my journey more livable than I would have thought possible and as enjoyable as circumstances allowed. I'm sure I would have received excellent care from one of the other many fine nurses at Northwest Georgia Oncology, but I believe Donna was especially handpicked by God to strengthen my heart, raise my spirits, and help get me through this difficult journey. ❧

TEACHING MOMENT:

I swear, I felt like just having Donna as my nurse did me almost as much good as the chemotherapy.

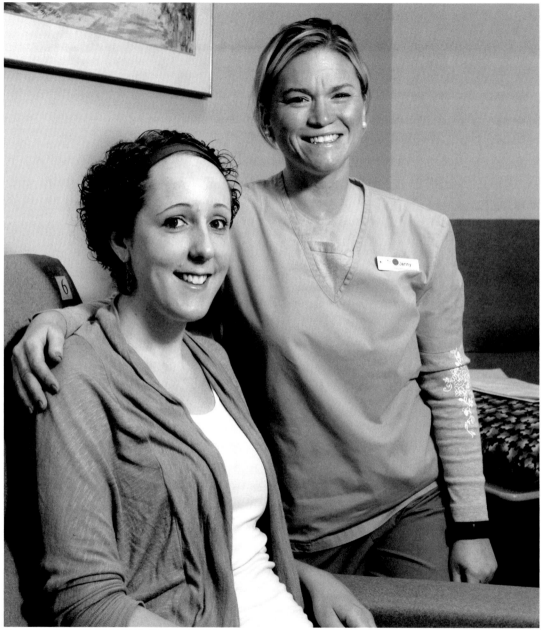

Jennifer Jamison, RN, BSN [right] with Grace Wright

What Pulls You Through

JENNIFER JAMISON, RN, BSN [MAINE CENTER FOR CANCER MEDICINE IN SCARBOROUGH, MAINE]

WRITTEN BY GRACE WRIGHT

SINCE MY CANCER diagnosis, I have been fortunate to meet the most supportive and caring group of people in every doctor's office and on every hospital visit. I have been constantly amazed at how compassionate almost every person has been, and I really believe that oncology calls for the most incredible personalities.

HOWEVER, there is one person who stands out as the shining light throughout my entire cancer journey—my treatment nurse, Jenny.

To say that Jenny embodies everything that an oncology nurse should be would be an understatement. Not only has she exceeded my expectations as a nurse, but at a time in my life when I needed a friend and someone to turn to in my most vulnerable moments, she's been there. Every time that I've hit a rough spot or wanted to give up, Jenny has been the one who's picked me up and helped me push forward. She's been the friend who "gets it" when no one else does.

There are a few moments that really stand out. One of these was my first day of chemotherapy—I was the last person in the treatment room that day, and as my last bag was finishing up, another nurse came over and offered to stay so that Jenny could go home—it was after 5 p.m. on a Friday, and Jenny had plans to go to a friend's housewarming party. Jenny refused and told the other nurse that she would stay with me until I was done. Then she sat down across from me and said, "I think housewarming parties are overrated anyway."

Another moment was the night when she only had a few minutes to check in with me at the hospital. I had such a rough day that she put everything else in her life on hold and spent an hour talking to me until I was calm enough to fall asleep. I remember sending her a message after having to do a few treatments without her because of conflicting schedules. I told her I didn't think I could do it without her—she was there for the next treatment and promised me she wouldn't go anywhere until I was done. She's been there for every one since then. Then there was the day after my birthday when I went in for treatment, and she had a birthday card on my chair in which she reminded me to celebrate another year and to look forward to many more—words that have often been used, but never had more meaning.

Looking forward to seeing her every other week, counting on her to check in with me on my hardest days, knowing that she'll be there if I need to talk, and knowing that because of cancer I've met my hero—these have made all the difference. People often tell me they are amazed that I'm still so optimistic and able to live life as any other 20-something would. I just smile every time and think how fortunate I am to have met Jenny—I know I wouldn't be here without her. I can't possibly explain it to people who haven't been in the same position, but I know that she's the reason I still have my life and my optimism—she has forced me to hang on tight in the times I really didn't have much in me to hold on to.

How do you thank someone for saving your life? In cancer, there's a lot of focus on survival. Physical survival, that is. It's easy to lose sight of the other kind of survival—being able to live day to day, to still dream as if you're going to live forever, to do something every day that you love, and to maintain some kind of normalcy. My doctors have saved my physical body, but Jenny really saved my life.

No matter how many times I thank her, I'm afraid she'll never really know that I'm just as thankful for her as I am for my doctors. It takes both parts of life to truly survive, especially at 25, when I've got a lot of living to do and lots of dreams to chase. I'm very proud to say that, after what has been the fight of my life, I've come out with both my physical body and a life that may be better than it was when I began.

But, I didn't do it alone, and while I embrace that feeling now, as I reflect on my journey, I am reminded how hard it was, and how it was Jenny who was there for me at every turn, reminding me that I had a life to live and had a lot to live for.

There's so much more to surviving cancer than coming out alive physically. We have to battle through so many obstacles that challenge our lives, our futures, and the dreams we're chasing. Without someone to pull us through all the things that doctors and medicine can't, we all need a hero—a hero like Jenny. ❧

My Hero

CHERYL ANN VALLEY, BSN, RN, CPON [CHILDREN'S HOSPITAL AT PROVIDENCE IN ANCHORAGE, ALASKA]

WRITTEN BY MORGAN TREON (AGE 14)

A HERO IS someone you can look up to and trust, someone who makes a difference in a person's life. Everyone has a hero, someone who changed her life for the better. My hero is Cheryl Ann Valley, my oncology nurse from the Children's Hospital of the King's Daughters (CHKD) because she is brave, wise, and caring.

THE DEFINITION OF brave is without fear, having or showing courage in the face of danger. My hero fits this definition of brave. Every year around St. Patrick's Day, there is an event called St. Baldrick's. People raise money for childhood cancer research by shaving their heads. My oncology nurse had long, beautiful hair but shaved it all off to raise research money—another example of Cheryl Ann's brave nature. An I.V. is used to put chemotherapy into the veins of the cancer patient. Cheryl Ann had to find a good vein and insert the I.V. into my vein. If she missed the vein, I would be in trouble and have chemo burn when I received chemotherapy. If I received too much chemo, I had the possibility of dying. Cheryl Ann gave me the powerful drugs through my I.V. If something went wrong, it would be her fault. She had to be brave when giving me the cure for my cancer.

When you are wise, you know a lot and know what to do in a situation. Cheryl Ann knew what drugs to give me and how much. She also knew what to do when someone was in trouble. My hero is wise because of her years in school. It's not easy to remember everything about childhood cancer; you also have to be wise and know when to use your knowledge.

CHKD was where I went to become cancer-free. Every time I arrived at the oncology clinic, I was greeted with a hug as warm as the sun from Cheryl Ann. Throughout the day, she would give hugs to try to make my visit better. She cared about how the cancer patient's visit was going. She always checked in on you and tried to make you comfy. If you asked her to do a craft with you, she'd stop and do a craft. My hero was always eager to please everyone at the CHKD oncology clinic.

My hero, the person I look up to, whom I trust, the person who changed my life in a good way and gave me hope in one of my darkest times is oncology nurse Cheryl Ann Valley. She is and always will be my hero because she's brave, wise, and caring. ❦

TEACHING MOMENT:

She cared about how the cancer patient's visit was going. She always checked in on you and tried to make you comfy. If you asked her to do a craft with you, she'd stop and do a craft.

The Next Best Thing

DIANE NECHI-FREGASSI, RN, BSN, OCN [HIGHLAND PARK HOSPITAL, KELLOGG CANCER CENTER IN HIGHLAND PARK, ILLINOIS]   WRITTEN BY TRACEY LANG

ON JULY 1, 2005, I was diagnosed with breast cancer at age 31. Little did I know just how much my life would change after my diagnosis. Everyone who is diagnosed with cancer is hoping for some kind of miracle, and if they have the privilege of getting Diane Nechi-Fregassi as their oncology nurse, they will soon learn that a miracle has come their way.

ANYONE WHO has to embark on a journey in "cancer land" needs someone who listens, understands, and truly cares. They need a caregiver who puts the person and not just the patient first, and that person is Diane. She has been on this journey with many people—those who have been taken by the horrors of cancer and those who are now survivors. She treats each of the people in her care as the only one whose life she is trying to save that day. She never rushes anyone or anything that she does, and somehow Diane always seems to score the best chemo room. Her nurse's coat is adorned with pins she has been awarded; these stem from the many people who've taken time to make certain the hospital knows just how top-notch Diane's patients think she is. Diane is not just a light at the end of the tunnel; she is the light that illuminates the entire journey.

Diane knows just how to navigate each road that a cancer patient travels, and those roads do not end once the person's treatment is done. When Diane becomes a part of your journey, she never pulls over and gets out. She is there to offer her expertise and answer any medical questions asked—to give emotional support (sharing in tears, anger, and joy). She knows when to hold your hand and just how tight to squeeze when she hugs you. And she knows how to be an advocate for her patients, just to name a few aspects of her job. Throughout treatment, as we are poked, prodded, filled with poison, awaiting blood work, and so on, there is no need to

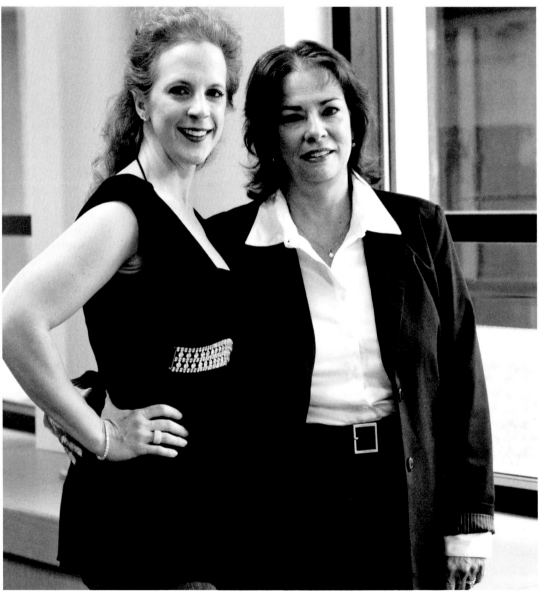

Diane Nechi-Fragassi, RN, BSN, OCN [right] with Tracey Lang

ask for anything, because when Diane is your nurse, she is on top of everything, providing answers to all of the questions you planned to ask and even some you had not realized you wanted answers to. If anyone is meant to be working in their field, Diane is meant to be an oncology nurse—and lucky me for that!

As a young woman with breast cancer, I was not the type of patient Diane sees on a regular basis. We are a rarer "breed," though we are growing in number. Breast cancer in young women tends to be more aggressive and does not fit into the statistics that most people are aware of. I came in armed with as much information as I could find, voicing how I wanted things handled and advocating for myself. When I first met Diane, I told her that she must have drawn the short straw that day. Diane kindly smiled, looking directly at me. As I looked back into her caring eyes, I saw a kind soul and immediately knew I was in the presence of an amazing woman. Diane embraced my personality and attitude toward fighting this disease. She is an integral and invaluable asset to me, a colonel and a soldier in my fight. I tell people all of the time that Diane rocks and everyone should be lucky enough to have Diane in their life!

No one is more on top of a patient's care than Diane. She works far too hard and too late. Even years after my chemotherapy has ended, my phone will ring at 7:30 on a Friday night, and the voice on the other end will be Diane. She calls simply to see how I am doing because she's thinking of me. She calls because she is aware that I have not been in for a while and wants to make sure I will be coming in soon. She calls because she genuinely cares. In return, I stop by the cancer center to see her because I love her and because seeing the warmth and sparkle in Diane's eyes and smile is an instant pick-me-up. There have been numerous times when I have been in random waiting rooms overhearing someone raving about their nurse, and then I find out they are speaking about my Diane. Needless to say, I am not surprised.

I never picked cancer—no one does. Cancer comes into people's lives with the agenda to destroy. Little does cancer know that when one woman named Diane is on the team of people trying to defeat it, her compassion and her help are incredibly powerful. Cancer is not a gift; however, I received one of the most amazing gifts because of cancer, and that is Diane. I can't imagine my life without her, and because of Diane being who she is and being so amazing at what she does, I have a life. A cancer diagnosis is not always the worst thing that can happen. Diane is not only an extraordinary healer but an extraordinary human being. Until there's a cure, there's the next best thing—Diane! ❧

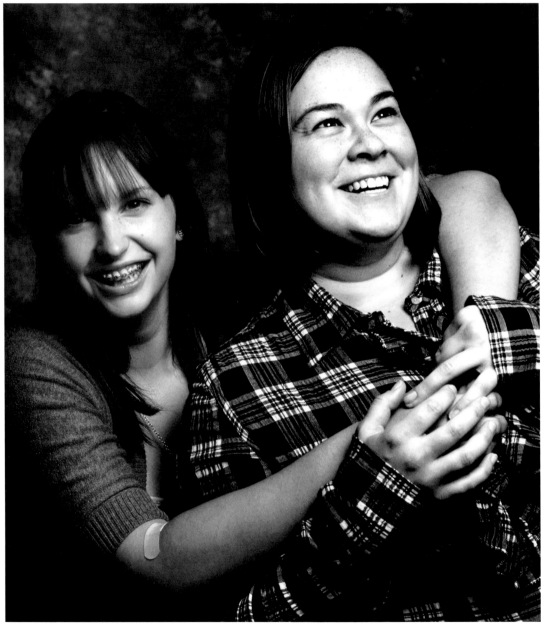

Jillian Wawrzynek, RN, OCN [right] with Sonia Whitman

My Hope and Inspiration

JILLIAN WAWRZYNEK, RN, OCN [PENNSYLVANIA ONCOLOGY HEMATOLOGY ASSOCIATES IN PHILADELPHIA, PENNSYLVANIA] WRITTEN BY SONIA WHITMAN

CANCER IS NEVER an easy journey. Countless surgeries, numerous blood draws, and so many medications, your head spins just trying to name them all. Cancer is easy for no one, whether you're a child, a mother, a father, or a grandparent. But it's just a little bit harder when you're a teenage girl.

IT WAS the summer before my freshman year. I had just turned 14. Overnight, I went from a spirited, carefree teenager to a teenager stricken with cancer and living in the hospital. It was traumatic. During what was supposed to be one of the most pivotal times in my life, I was living it all away from comfort in a hospital.

I had osteosarcoma, a form of bone cancer. I endured six rounds of high-dose chemotherapy, a knee replacement, various catheterizations, and countless other procedures that only live in nightmares. Before I knew it, I found myself spiraling deep into depression. There was no light at the end of the tunnel. I had a one-way ticket on a high-speed train—estimated time of arrival unknown, destination unknown.

I was five months into treatment and one month into depression (although it felt like centuries) when I met Bean—or rather, nurse Jillian. At the time, Bean was an eight-year survivor of osteosarcoma. She had been cured right on that very floor of the hospital, using the same medications, techniques, and even doctors.

We met sometime in January 2008. I was in the hospital for a routine blood transfusion. When I got settled in my room, I found out my nurse for that day would be Jill. I'd heard of her but never met her, which was something I was looking forward to. Jill spent hours with me that day talking to me about everything she endured when she was sick. She even told me about the time her stepdad had to drag her out of the house to get chemo. Instantly, we shared a bond, although I never had to be dragged out of the house. We sat and talked about everything: life before chemo, life after chemo, medications, and effects the chemotherapy had on our bodies. For hours, it was just two young girls talking.

Later that day, my doctor came in to check on me and took my mom out in the hall. He asked my mom, "What happened to Sonia? She has improved emotionally and mentally so much since I saw her yesterday." My mom simply replied, "Jill."

Jill would go on to be my source of hope until I finished chemo in March 2008. She is still my source of hope, and it's been two years since I finished chemo. She's helped me with everything from post-chemo care to being a normal teenager again. She's helped me on my return to sports, return to school, and return to life.

Jill is more than just a caregiver to me. Jill is my nurse. Jill is my friend. Jill is my big sister. Jill is my hero. Jill is my inspiration. Jill is my hope. Without Jill cheering me on, I don't know where I'd be today.

I saw the way Jill helped me when I was sick, and it hit something within me. I was so moved by what she did for me that I decided to be the next Jill. I'm currently exploring careers in nursing. I will have my certified nursing assistance degree in a year when I graduate high school. After that, it's off to nursing school for me. Without Jill, I don't know where I'd be. ❧

TEACHING MOMENT:

Jill is more than just a caregiver to me. Jill is my nurse. Jill is my friend. Jill is my big sister. Jill is my hero. Jill is my inspiration. Jill is my hope.

A Return Visit

ANN BELL, RN, OCN [WHIDBEY GENERAL HOSPITAL IN COUPEVILLE, WASHINGTON]

WRITTEN BY DENNIS WISCHMEIER

IN AUGUST 2005, I was 28 years old and married with an amazing 3-year-old daughter. My wife and I were expecting our second child, and I had a great job flying for the U.S. Navy as a Naval Flight Officer. Then, in the middle of a routine week, I was diagnosed with stage 3 testicular cancer. It had metastasized into an 11-centimeter tumor in my abdomen. Shortly thereafter, I met nurse Ann.

WHILE SHE is not a cancer survivor, she is the closest a nonsurvivor can get to sympathizing with a patient. Her energetic attitude and support to a scared patient, his young daughter, and pregnant wife deserve awards. Her connection to me went far beyond her prior military experience and having her own young child. Working in the oncology ward was not a step to another position—it was her desire from the beginning and her passion after she left the military and put herself through school.

My first week at the hospital was the most physically painful because I did not have a port. With my difficult veins, it took multiple "attempts" to get the metal "telephone pole" jabbed into my arm. All the while, Ann was there to give me breaks and entertain my family. It is a rare individual who can quickly understand the real need within hours of an introduction. The doctor diagnosed me, but the nurses physically cured me.

After I had my port installed, I felt the chemo effects slowly build up and followed every word that Ann gave me. In the meantime, our focus was split between my treatment and planning a C-section for the birth of our son around my chemo rounds. Ann recognized the challenges that this brought both mentally and physically on my wife and me, going out of her way to talk about her family and open herself up to us. She gave a personal touch to everything. Every blood test report, every white blood cell booster shot, every wipe of the

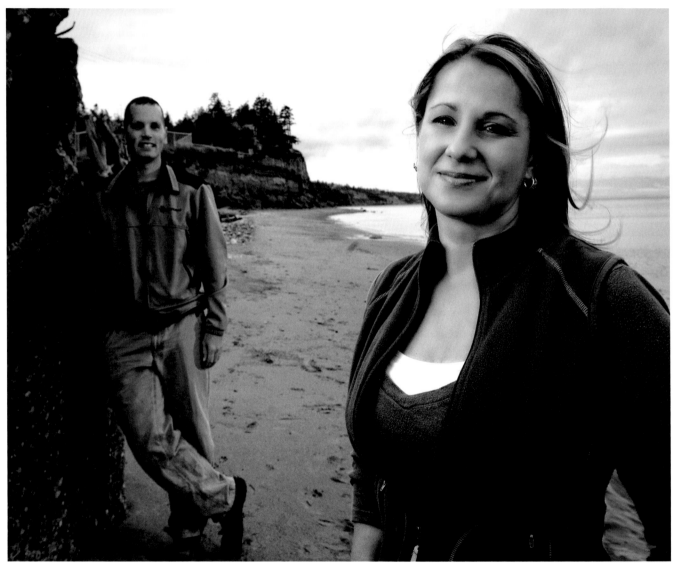

Ann Bell, RN, OCN [front] with Dennis Wischmeier

numbing solution over my port, every reminder to chew gum prior to the flushing of my port—was preceded by the reminder of why I was going through it.

Then, between my second and third round of chemo, my son Ethan entered the world. Words cannot express how I longed to have all the focus on my beautiful wife, newborn son, and toddler daughter. Everyone, from the hospital staff to our family and friends, would eye the four of us with joy and sympathy. I was too weak to stand for long periods of time and could not hold my newborn son for extended periods of time. While sitting at my wife's hospital bed, I had to have family help me remember when to take my drugs.

For the first time in months, I was fighting anger at my circumstances. Ann knew this while all the staff at the oncology ward congratulated me on the birth of our child. Ann's passion for being intentional is something that will never leave our memory. When we brought our brand-new baby into the oncology ward, once again, Ann spearheaded the effort to rush at us, loudly, with tears, and put all the focus on my wife and baby. I remember being there physically but mentally looking back from afar thinking that it was a perfect moment—the focus was finally on them (even if we were all in the oncology ward)!

After my last and most physically demanding round of chemo, Ann was there as my doctor told me the tumor had not dissipated as desired and that my blood tumor markers did not drop to the rock-bottom level they wanted. I was to undergo a major surgery, retroperitoneal lymph node dissection, to rid me of the tumor and surrounding lymph nodes. After my oncologist left, Ann swooped in, held my hands, looked me right in the eye, and said, "This is a good thing. Remember this. You will survive; you've won. Recuperate. Enjoy your family and the holidays. [My surgery was planned for January 4, 2006.] Call me anytime at home or work. I wish all my patients were like you." Then she just sat there, frozen, like I was.

I am now a four-year cancer survivor. I am still in the Navy and keep in touch with Ann as often as I can. She said something to me during a visit that shocked me: "We hardly get a survivor back in to visit us!" When she told me this, I told her, "I never forget thinking about you, and thanking God for you. And believe me when I say that while others are not flooding the spaces to thank you, they too are thinking the same thing." I think she knows this, but everyone can use encouragement, and Ann and the rest of the staff definitely do not get enough of it. To all survivors out there—thank your oncology nurses today!   ❧

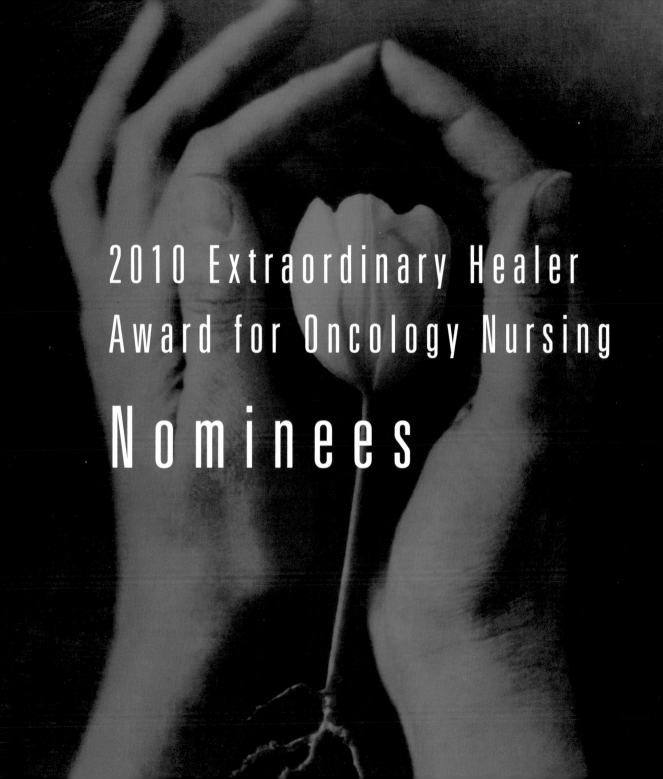

2010 Extraordinary Healer
Award for Oncology Nursing

Nominees

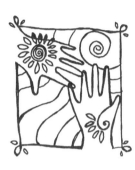

CURE congratulates each nurse who was nominated. You are all extraordinary healers.

Carla Alling, RN, OCN / Arizona Oncology

Benita Austin, MSN, ANP-BC / Barnes-Jewish Hospital

Patti Barkley, RN, MS, ANP-C / M.D. Anderson Cancer Center

Dawn Barringer, RN, BSN / Cancer Centers of North Carolina

Karen Bechtol, RN, OCN / Gynecologic Oncology Associates of Orange County

Michelle Beil, RN, BS, OCN / White Plains Hospital Center

Ann Bell, RN, OCN / Whidbey General Hospital & Clinics

Peggy Beltz, RN, CPON / Children's Hospitals and Clinics of Minnesota

Annie Bloomquist, RN / Wind River Oncology, Riverton Memorial Hospital

Janell Bontrager, RN, BSN / Goshen General Hospital

Vadim Borchenko, RN, OCN / Tower Hematology Oncology Medical Group

Martha Boyle, RN, BSN, OCN / Texas Oncology

Susan Brandt, RN / UPMC Shadyside Hospital

Amy Brassard, RN, MS, OCN / Zimmer Cancer Center, New Hanover Regional Medical Center

Sharon Braswell, RN, OCN / Birmingham Hematology-Oncology Associates

Robin Brendel, BSN, OCN / Memorial Sloan-Kettering Cancer Center

Sue Brillheart, RN / Connecticut Oncology & Hematology

Sharon Britain, RN, CACP, OCN / Memorial Health System Cancer Center

Jackie Broadway-Duren, MSN, FNP-BC / M.D. Anderson Cancer Center

Sharon Brogan, RN, OCN / Lankenau Hospital

Amy Brown, RN / Johns Hopkins Hospital

Christy Brown, RN, BSN / Indiana University Simon Cancer Center

Meg Brown, RN, OCN / Seattle Cancer Care Alliance

Donna Bush, RN, OCN / Northwest Georgia Oncology Center

Sandra Canty, RN, MS, OCN / Elmhurst Memorial Center for Health

Mary Carroll, RN, BSN, OCN / City of Hope

Cheryl Casella-Rymer, ARNP-BC / Palm Beach Institute of Hematology & Oncology

Patricia Charles, RN, BSN / Colorado Hematology & Oncology

Ron Chubin, RN, OCN / Shady Grove Adventist Hospital

Leslie Collis-Clarke, ARNP-C / James A. Haley VA Hospital

Pattie Conroy-Vatalaro, RN, BSN, OCN / On Care Hawaii

Maryrose Custer, RN / Richard A. Henson Cancer Center

Penny Daugherty, RN, MS, OCN / Southeastern Gynecologic Oncology

Linda David, RN / Smilow Cancer Hospital at Yale-New Haven

April Davis, RN / Cancer Center of the Carolinas

Doreen DePalmo, RN, MS / Saint Margaret Mercy's Oncology Center

Vicki Doctor, RN, OCN, BSN, BSW / CTCA at Western Regional Medical Center

Emily Fagan, RN / Monroe Carell Jr. Children's Hospital at Vanderbilt

Amy Fair, RN / Simmons Firm

Karolina Faysman, RN, MSN, NP / UCLA Medical Center

Leeanne Fenney, RN / Baystate Medical Center

Gena Fetch, RN, BSN, OCN / Cancer Care Northwest

Kathy Fetherolf, RN, OCN / Morgan Hospital & Medical Center

Patricia Frilot-Mitchell, RN / Texas Oncology

Shelley Frohm, RN, BSN, OCN / Utah Cancer Specialists

Mary Gaffney, RN / Oncology Hematology Associates of Southwest Indiana

Susan Gandley, RN, BSN, OCN / Mercy San Juan Medical Center

Joan Gibble, MS, ARNP / Florida Cancer Specialists

Mary Gleason, BSN, OCN / South Shore Hematology-Oncology Associates

Annette Graham, ANP, AOCNP / Virginia Cancer Institute

Mary Grande, RN, OCN / Roger Williams Medical Center

Coveny Greco, RN, OCN / Cancer Centers of North Carolina

Clarice Grens, RN / VA Connecticut Healthcare System

Margaret Griffin, RN / Dana-Farber/Brigham & Women's Cancer Center at Faulkner Hospital

Irene Haapoja, RN, MS, AOCN / Rush University Medical Center

Susan Halbritter, CNP, MS, ANP-BC, AOCN / Sanford Cancer Center Hematology & Oncology

Kim Haley, RN, BSN / Crescent City Physicians

Jean Hall, RN / Allegheny General Hospital

Nancy Harold, RN / National Cancer Insitute

Ronald Heiser, RN / Hernando-Pasco Hospice

Deborah Henry-LaVigne, RN / Highland Radiation Oncology, University of Rochester Medical Center

Kassy Hetzel, RN, BSN / Children's Hospital of Wisconsin

Jan Hildebrant, RN / Surrey Memorial Hospital

Marie Holleman, RN / Texas Oncology

Sandra Holt, RN, OCN / University of Maryland Medical Center

Vickie Hutchens, RN / Cancer Specialist of Oklahoma

Denise Ives, RN, BSN / Cleveland Clinic

Jennifer Jamison, RN, BSN / Maine Center for Cancer Medicine & Blood Disorders

Elizabeth Jasper, RN / Jewish Hospital

Mary Jerome, RN / UAB Comprehensive Cancer Center

Gabriela Kaplan, RN, MSN, AOCN / Care Alternative Hopsice

Megan Jane Keast, RN / Jimmy Everest Center for Cancer and Blood Disorders in Children, Oklahoma University Medical Center

Nancy Keegan, RN, BA, OCN / Hematology-Oncology Associates of Central New York

Ivy Kelley, RN / Shands at the University of Florida

Janelle Kerns, RN, OCN / Iowa Cancer Specialists

David Makumi Kinyanjui, RN / Aga Khan University Hospital

Melanie Kirksey, RN, BSN, OCN / Texas Oncology

Loraye Klamm, RN, BSN, OCN / Rocky Mountain Cancer Centers

Molly Knigge, MS, CCC-SLP, BRS-S / The University of Wisconsin Voice and Swallowing Clinic

Mitch Ladyman, RN / Texas Oncology

Priscilla Lawrence, MSN, NP-C / Lynn Cancer Institute, Boca Raton Community Hospital

Carol Leonard, RN / Pitt County Memorial Hospital

Carol Lieban, RN, BSN, OCN / Queen's Medical Center

ChiaChun Lu, RN, OCN / Cancer Institute of New Jersey

Riza Lumauag, RN, BSN / Progressive Care

Joanna Lupardus, RN, BSN, OCN / Marietta Memorial Hospital

Anne Luptrawan, MSN, FNP / Cedars-Sinai Medical Center

Julie Lutz, APN, FNP-BC, MS, OCN / University of Chicago
Hospitals

Janet Mack, RN, OCN / Aroostook Medical Center

Rita Mack, RN, BSN / Vitas Innovative Hospice Care

Arla Martin, RN / South Orange County Hematology
Oncology Associates

Julie Mattison-Chad, RN, BSN / Gynecologic Oncology
Associates

Lana McCallum, RN, BSN, MS, ANP, CRNI, AOCN / Greeley
Medical Clinic

Margaret McMullin, MSN, APRN, BC, AOCNP / Dana-Farber
Cancer Institute

Julie McNelis, RN, OCN, CRNI / Alvin & Lois Lapidus Cancer
Institute, Sinai Hospital

Mioara Miok, RN / South Macomb Internists

Jessica Mitchell, RN, MSN, NP, MPH / Mayo Clinic

Machelle Moeller, RN, MSN, CNP, OCN / Cleveland Clinic

Dana Monroe, RN, OCN / San Francisco Oncology
Associates

Joyce Montgomery, RMTP / Crossroads Meeting House

Anne Monticelli, RN, BSN, OCN / Lash Group,
AmerisourceBergen Specialty Group

Lori Anne Morrow, RN, BSN, OCN / Palmetto Hematology
Oncology, Spartanburg Regional Healthcare

Susan Nasif, RN, MSN, APNP / Froedtert & The Medical
College of Wisconsin

Diane Nechi-Fragassi, RN, BSN, OCN / Kellogg Cancer
Center, Highland Park Hospital

Barbara Nichols, RT / Presbyterian Hospital of Rockwall

Barbara Perchalski, RN / Chattanooga Gyn-Oncology

Noemie Pouliot, RN / Thomas Jefferson University Hospital

Tina Pryor, RN, BSN, OCN / Virginia Oncology Associates

Michelle Ramirez, RN, OCN / Texas Oncology

Paula Richardson, BSN, OCN / Samaritan Ambulatory
Infusion Center

Samantha Rippetoe, RN, BSN, OCN / Vanderbilt-Ingram
Cancer Center

Barbara Rogers, CRNP, MN, AOCN, ANP-BC / Fox Chase
Cancer Center

Kathy Rothering, RN, BSN / University of Wisconsin
Hospitals and Clinics

Mari Rude, RN, ANP, AOCN / Lester and Sue Smith Breast
Center, Baylor College of Medicine

Karen Ruppert, RN / Roswell Park Cancer Institute

Andrea Russell, RN, BSN, BHN / Carson City Hospital

Renee Sarnicki, RN / Rahway Regional Cancer Center

Cynthia Schuster, RN / Cancer Care Specialists of Central
Illinois

Melinda Shaw, RN, OCN / Redwood Regional Medical Group

Wanda Shehan, RN, OCN / Sentara Potomac Hospital

Melissa Shelby, ACNP-C, RN, BSN, OCN / Johns Hopkins
Bayview Medical Center

Jaime Smith, RN, BSN, OCN / Perry County Memorial
Hospital

Becky Stewart, RN / Legacy Good Samaritan Hospital

Bonnie Strudas, RN, BSN, OCN / Massachusetts General
Hospital

Pamela Tabler, RN, MS, BSN, CHPN / Joliet Area
Community Hospice

Sharon Thacker, RN / Huntington Hospital

Jacquie Toia, DNP, RN, MS / Children's Memorial Hospital

Ellen Tolentino, RN, BSN, OCN / Baylor Charles A.
Sammons Cancer Center

Karen Tooker, RN, BSN / Office of Steven Vogl, MD

Lori Travis, RN / Geisinger Cancer Center

Cheryl Ann Valley, RN, BSN, CPON / Children's Hospital at
Providence

Daniel VanderGast, RN, BSN / Greater Philadelphia Cancer
and Hematology Specialists

Dorothy Wahrman, RN, OCN / Nebraska Cancer Specialists

Melissa Walker, APNP, AOCN / ProHealth Care Regional
Cancer Center

Dawn Warren, RN / St. Vincent's East Hospital

Jillian Wawrzynek, RN, OCN / Pennsylvania Oncology
Hematology Associates

Carei Weedham-Wells, RN / Office of Guillermo Abesada-
Terk, MD

Matt Wendel, RN / Office of Jeffrey Templer, MD

Ann Werle, RN, BSN, CBCN / Covenant Breast Health
Center

Darlene Williams, LVN / Arlington Cancer Center

Rachel Williamson, RN / North Mississippi Medical Center

Carolanne Wismer, RN, OCN / Fox Chase Cancer Center

Carol Woodcock, RN, OCN / Glenda Tanner Vasicek Cancer
Treatment Center

Kathryn Carlson Wrammert, MSN, APRN-BC, WHNP-BC /
Winship Cancer Institute of Emory University

Kathy Zanatto, RN / Valley Medical Oncology Consultants

Mandie Zerka, RN, OCN / Genesys Hurley Cancer Institute